This book is due for return on or before the last date shown below.

16. DEC. 199

Don Gresswell Ltd., London, N.21 Cat. No. 1208   DG 02242/71

00001381

ENTERED

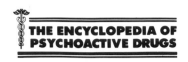
THE ENCYCLOPEDIA OF PSYCHOACTIVE DRUGS

IN 25 VOLUMES
Each title on a specific drug or drug-related problem

OVER-THE-COUNTER DRUGS

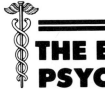

THE ENCYCLOPEDIA OF PSYCHOACTIVE DRUGS

OVER-THE-COUNTER DRUGS

Harmless or Hazardous?

PAUL SANBERG, Ph.D.

Ohio University

RICHARD M. T. KREMA

Ohio University

GENERAL EDITOR (U.S.A.)
Professor Solomon H. Snyder, M.D.

*Distinguished Service Professor of
Neuroscience, Pharmacology, and Psychiatry at
The Johns Hopkins University School of Medicine*

GENERAL EDITOR (U.K.)
Professor Malcolm H. Lader, D.Sc., Ph.D., M.D., F.R.C. Psych.

*Professor of Clinical Psychopharmacology
at the Institute of Psychiatry, University of London,
and Honorary Consultant to the Bethlem Royal and Maudsley Hospitals*

Burke Publishing Company Limited
LONDON

Acknowledgements
Photos courtesy of Bayer AG, The Bettmann Archive, Inc., Library of
Congress, National Library of Medicine, Julie Nichols, Susan Quist, UPI/Bettmann
Newsphotos.

CIP data
Sanberg, Paul
   Over-the-counter drugs – (Encyclopedia of psychoactive drugs)
   1. Drugs, Nonprescription
   1. Title   II. Krema, Richard M.T.
   III. Series
   615'1   RM671.A1
ISBN 0 222 01455 5 Hardbound
ISBN 0 222 01456 3 Paperback

Burke Publishing Company Limited
Pegasus House, 116-120 Golden Lane, London EC1Y 0TL, England.
Typeset in England by Datatrend, Hull.
Printed in Spain, by Jerez Industrial, S.A.

CONTENTS

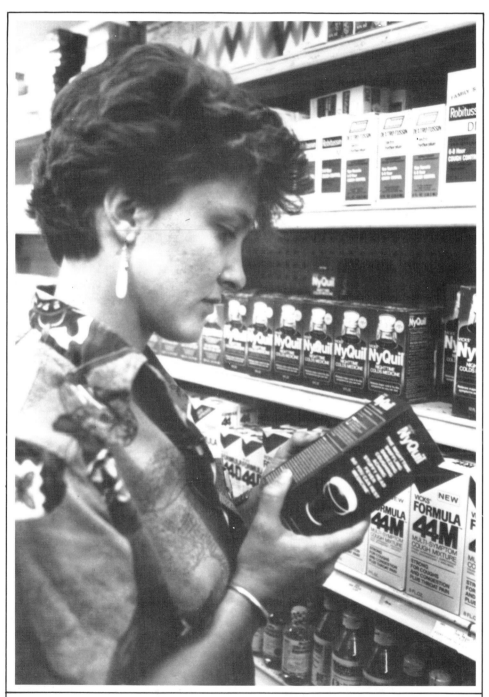

A careful consumer studies the label on a package of nonprescription medicine. Many shoppers mistakenly assume that all preparations available without a doctor's prescription are safe.

INTRODUCTION

The late twentieth century has seen the rapid growth of both the legitimate medical use and the illicit, non-medical abuse of an increasing number of drugs which affect the mind. Both use and abuse are very high in general in the United States of America and great concern is voiced there. Other Western countries are not far behind and cannot afford to ignore the matter or to shrug off the consequent problems. Nevertheless, differences between countries may be marked and significant: they reflect such factors as social habits, economic status, attitude towards the young and towards drugs, and the ways in which health care is provided and laws are enacted and enforced.

Drug abuse particularly concerns the young but other age groups are not immune. Alcoholism in middle-aged men and increasingly in middle-aged women is one example, tranquillizers in women another. Even the old may become alcoholic or dependent on their barbiturates. And the most widespread form of addiction, and the one with the most dire consequences to health, is cigarette-smoking.

Why do so many drug problems start in the teenage and even pre-teenage years? These years are critical in the human life-cycle as they involve maturation from child to adult. During these relatively few years, adolescents face the difficult task of equipping themselves physically and intellectually for adulthood and of establishing goals that make adult life worthwhile while coping with the search for personal identity, assuming their sexual roles and learning to come to terms with authority. During this intense period of growth

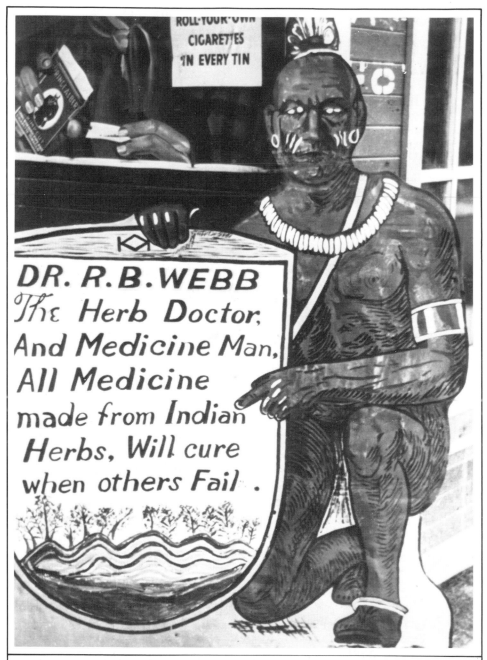

Medicines made from herbs and other plant substances were widely used in the 18th and 19th centuries, but gradually synthesized drugs gained in popularity. Since the 1960s, however, herbal-remedy use has increased.

and activity, bewilderment and conflict are inevitable, and peer pressure to experiment and to escape from life's apparent problems becomes overwhelming. Drugs are increasingly available and offer a tempting respite.

Unfortunately, the consequences may be serious. But the penalties for drug-taking must be put into perspective. Thus, addicts die from heroin addiction but people also die from alcoholism and even more from smoking-related diseases. Also, one must separate the direct effects of drug-taking from those indirectly related to the life-style of so many addicts. The problems of most addicts include many factors other than drug-taking itself. The chaotic existence or social deterioration of some may be the cause rather than the effect of drug abuse.

Drug use and abuse must be set into its social context. It reflects a complex interaction between the drug substance (naturally-occurring or synthetic), the person (psychologically normal or abnormal), and society (vigorous or sick). Fads affect drug-taking, as with most other human activities, with drugs being heavily abused one year and unfashionable the next. Such swings also typify society's response to drug abuse. Opiates were readily available in European pharmacies in the last century but are stringently controlled now. Marijuana is accepted and alcohol forbidden in many Islamic countries; the reverse obtains in most Western countries.

The use of psychoactive drugs dates back to prehistory. Opium was used in Ancient Egypt to alleviate pain and its main constituent, morphine, remains a favoured drug for pain relief. Alcohol was incorporated into religious ceremonies in the cradles of civilization in the Near and Middle East and has been a focus of social activity ever since. Coca leaf has been chewed by the Andean Indians to lessen fatigue; and its modern derivative, cocaine, was used as a local anaesthetic. More recently, a succession of psychoactive drugs have been synthesized, developed and introduced into medicine to allay psychological distress and to treat psychiatric illness. But, even so, these innovations may present unexpected problems, such as the difficulties in stopping the long-term use of tranquillizers or slimming-pills, even when taken under medical supervision.

The Encyclopedia of Psychoactive Drugs provides information about the nature of the effects on mind and body of

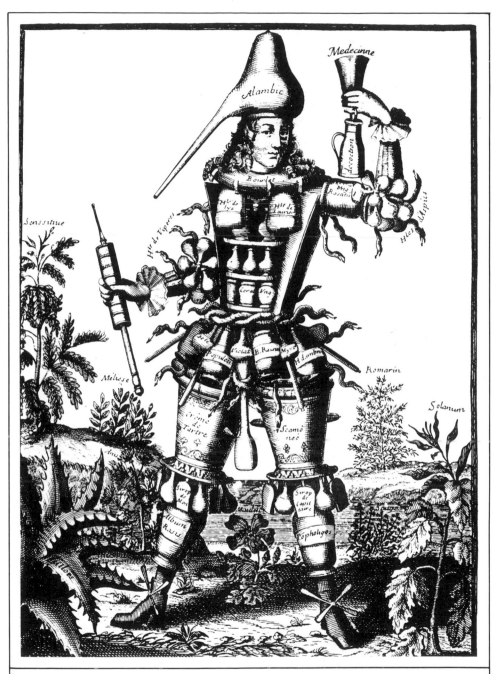

A French engraving portrays a 17th-century apothecary, or druggist, as a walking medicine cabinet. Societies all over the world have used and experimented with healing and mind-altering drugs since the beginning of recorded time. The Greeks, for example, had a form of aspirin 2,500 years ago, and marijuana was used medically as early as 3000 B.C.

alcohol and drugs and the possible results of abuse. Topics include where the drugs come from, how they are made, how they affect the body and how the body deals with these chemicals; the effects on the mind, thinking, emotions, the will and the intellect are detailed; the processes of use and abuse are discussed, as are the consequences for everyday activities such as school work, employment, driving, and dealing with other people. Pointers to identifying drug users and to ways of helping them are provided. In particular, this series aims to dispel myths about drug-taking and to present the facts as objectively as possible without all the emotional distortion and obscurity which surrounds the subject. We seek neither to exaggerate nor to play down the complex topics concerning various forms of drug abuse. We hope that young people will find answers to their questions and that others—parents and teachers, for example—will also find the series helpful.

The series was originally written for American readers by American experts. Often the problem with a drug is particularly pressing in the USA or even largely confined to that country. We have invited a series of British experts to adapt the series for use in non-American English-speaking countries and believe that this widening of scope has successfully increased the relevance of these books to take account of the international drug scene.

This volume deals with a wide variety of medicines which are available "over-the-counter" in chemists' shops and even more widely in general stores and supermarkets. These remedies are used for pain relief, to treat colds, and to provide mild stimulation and some help with anxiety and insomnia. Although in general these medicines are effective, safe and acceptable, some people find that their use of these drugs gets out of hand to the point of an abuse or dependence problem. The various drugs, their use, misuse and abuse, are described here, and some advice is given on how to cope with the problem. The book was written originally by Paul Sanberg and Richard Krema and has been modified extensively by Paul Williams of the Institute of Psychiatry, University of London.

M.H. Lader

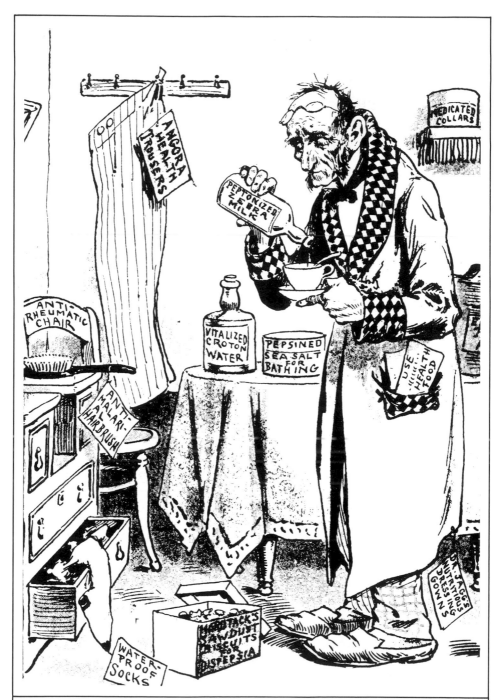

A health fanatic pours himself a cup of "peptonized zebra milk". Some products in the multimillion-dollar nutrition market are no more effective than those satirized in this magazine cartoon.

CHAPTER 1

THE DRUGGING OF THE WESTERN WORLD

Why should a person worry about taking a drug that can be purchased by anyone at the local pharmacy and without a prescription? What do aspirin and cough syrup, for example, have to do with drug abuse?

The general public has been led to assume that any drug made available without prescription has been thoroughly tested and is thus well established as safe and effective treatment for the ailment for which it is intended. In fact, the US Food and Drug Administration (FDA) has not found evidence that this assumption is true for many over-the-counter (OTC) products. The FDA's OTC advisory panels, established about ten years ago, have concluded that only approximately one-third of the ingredients in the 300,000 brands of OTC products available in America which they studied were safe and effective for their intended uses.

Evaluating the safety and effectiveness of a drug requires rigorous scientific testing. Strict scientific assessments of the ingredients in OTC products, based on "double-blind" studies (discussed in Chapter 6), were initiated in the early 1970s. They are designed to ensure that the drug's effects are real rather than imagined and that they could not be produced by a placebo—a substance, such as sugar, that produces no noticeable effects.

In a double-blind study only the experimenter, and neither the administrator of the drug nor the patient knows whether the ingested substance is a placebo or the actual drug. Therefore, the patient cannot know or be given any clues regarding the pill's actual content. If a statistically significant number of patients feel an effect no matter what is ingested, the experimenter can conclude that the "drug" is not effective. However, if the patient consistently notices an effect only when taking the drug, one can conclude that the drug is effective. Many of the approximately 500,000 OTC products, composed of 500 to 1,000 active ingredients, have not been studied in this fashion.

Many of the OTC products for which there is no proof of safety or efficacy do not present a serious health hazard for most people if taken in the recommended amounts and for the symptoms they are supposed to alleviate. But when these drugs are used in excess, or when they are used when they are not needed at all—and unfortunately this is the case for many people—they can become hazardous.

To understand fully a drug's hazards and potential for abuse, one must understand the drug itself. This book describes the available OTC drugs, and their potential dangers and adverse effects.

When drug abuse is mentioned one often thinks of a

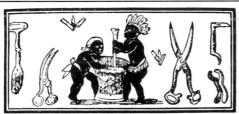

Good News to the Sick.

Veragainſt *Ludgate* Church, within *Black-Fryers* Gate-way, at *Lillies-Head*, Liveth your old Friend Dr. *Caſe*, who faithfully Cures the Grand P—, with all its Symptoms, very Cheap, Private, and without the leaſt Hindrance of Buſineſs. *Note*, He hath been a Phyſitian 33 Years, and gives Advice in any Diſtem per *gratis*.

All ye that are of *Venus* Race,
Apply your ſelves to Dr. *Caſe*;
Who, with a Box or two of PILLS,
Will ſoon remove your painfull ILLS.

A poster advertises the services of "Dr. Case", who was a notorious 18th-century quack. Prospective patients were assured that Dr. Case, "with a box or two of PILLS, will soon remove your painfull ILLS"—lines not very different from thosed used to advertise some of today's OTC drugs.

person who takes recreational drugs—such as marijuana, cocaine or heroin—to escape reality and get "high". However, drug abuse also includes the behaviour of a person who takes more medication than is recommended or required to alleviate aches and pains. In fact, this type of drug taking can be just as dangerous as using heroin. For example, aspirin is often used to commit suicide. Taking too much of any drug, no matter what the initial motivation, nonetheless constitutes abuse.

Today there is good reason to give this topic serious consideration. An ever-increasing number of people rely on one kind of OTC product or another just to get through the day. Several decades ago people showed a much higher degree of "frustration tolerance" than now and thus depended upon fewer drugs. Undoubtedly, part of the reason why they were able to put up with more aches and pains is that, in many cases, the drugs that could alleviate these symptoms were either not available or did not yet exist. Thus they did not have the expectation of "instant relief" which many have today. In addition, the volume of advertising was much smaller, and consequently people had com-

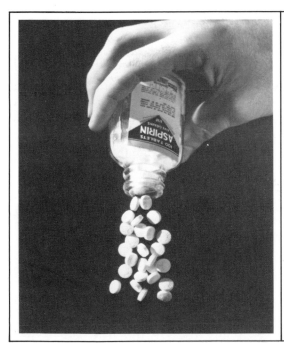

Aspirin is one of the most widely used OTC drugs. For most people it is a relatively safe, nonaddictive medication that effectively treats pain, fever and inflammation. For others, especially those who misuse it, aspirin can cause ringing in the ears, nausea, heartburn, vomiting, internal bleeding, convulsions and even death. More hospitalizations for adverse drug reactions are due to aspirin than to any other drug.

paratively little information on what kinds of products were available.

But the situation has changed. Now, people expect there to be a drug solution for every discomfort, from a hangover to cancer, and over the years we have been convinced that it is available from OTC products. Television commercials are especially effective, as are magazine and newspaper advertisements and the anecdotal evidence of family and friends.

When it comes to taking drugs, children follow examples set by their parents. A very large proportion of parents take OTC and other drugs on a daily basis. Several studies have concluded that what influences whether or not children go on to abuse drugs is not so much the type of drug the parents take but just the fact that they take drugs. Parental use of any type of drug (pills, alcohol or even coffee) tends to foster drug-taking in the children. And perhaps because child rearing has generally been the duty of the woman, a child is much more likely to take drugs if the mother, rather than the father, uses drugs.

In addition to relatives and friends, family doctors also regularly encourage the use of nonprescription drugs. A few years ago six hundred doctors participated in a study intended to evaluate the doctor's role in perpetuating OTC drug use. The results showed that physicians who were likely to prescribe prescription drugs also frequently recommended nonprescription (i.e., OTC) drugs.

People are overmedicated throughout the industrialized world. The average household stocks 17 different OTC products which they use to treat 70% of their illnesses. The results of a questionnaire published in 1983 showed that in any 30-week period approximately 85% of all families purchased at least one OTC drug. Table 1 shows the frequency with which people in America use OTC products. OTC drug manufacturers reported that between 1980 and 1981 there was a 12% increase in sales, and according to another report, published in September 1983, Americans annually spend somewhere between $4 billion and $8 billion on OTC products.

Case Study

Tammy was an exceptionally bright 15-year-old American high-school student. She had many friends and had had

Table 1

Frequency of OTC Use	
FREQUENCY	% OF 2558 TEST SUBJECTS
Very often	8.0
Occasionally	37.3
Not very often	45.4
Never	9.3

SOURCE: Adapted from Johnson, R.E. and Rope, C.R., "Health Status and Social Factors in Non-prescribed Drug Use," *Medical Care*, 21:225–233, 1983.

a steady boyfriend for almost two months. But in spite of constant reassurance from friends and family, she did not believe that she was pretty. Tammy was convinced that she was disgustingly fat, though her father told her that 131 pounds for a 5′ 8″ girl was quite normal, especially since she was still growing. But she wanted to become a model, and models are supposed to be skinny. Just thinking about her "condition" made her depressed for long periods. All efforts at dieting failed. One day her attention was captured by an advertisement that promised a quick and easy method to get rid of excess weight. By using an OTC aid, she could lose 10 pounds or more in a few weeks—guaranteed!

In the pharmacy she gazed at the colourful boxes of diet-aid products, her dreams of a modelling career seemingly within reach. Tammy chose an extra-strength brand. She succeeded in losing 11 pounds in sixteen days, but she regained the weight in the following week. She dieted again and managed to achieve her dream weight of 117 pounds, but this lasted for only two days. She tried other diet aids, by themselves and in various combinations, yet the pounds just would not stay off.

She began to have headaches and stomachaches, and often felt nauseous and irritable. The only time she had a good night's sleep was when she did not take her pills for a day or so. Then she began oversleeping and missing classes. The only way she was able to function at school or hold her weekend job was if she ingested up to five capsules at a time. Constantly irritable, Tammy finally lost her closest friends and gained the nickname "crabby Tammy".

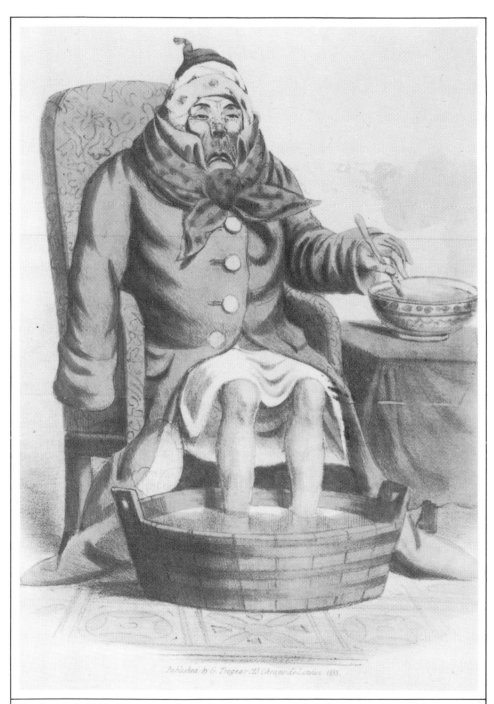

Only slightly less ancient than the common cold is the common-cold remedy. Here, an early 19th-century sufferer follows the medical advice of his day by soaking his feet and bundling up.

CHAPTER 2

COLD REMEDIES

An article recently published in an American medical journal told of a 23-year-old woman who decided to drink a full bottle, or 300 ml (millilitres), of Nyquil after she had run out of whisky. Nyquil, an OTC cold remedy sold in the USA, contains 25% alcohol and includes 6,000 mg (milligrams) of paracetamol (a pain reliever), 7.5 mg of doxylamine succinate (an antihistamine), 6 mg of ephedrine sulphate (a decongestant), and 15 mg of dextromethorphan hydrobromide (a cough suppressant). The recommended dose for a cold is 30 ml, or about two tablespoons. Therefore, the woman consumed ten times the recommended dose of this cold remedy. A few hours later after taking the Nyquil, the woman felt extremely nauseous and vomited repeatedly. Two days later she was admitted to a nearby hospital and diagnosed as having severe hepatitis and kidney failure.

Consuming cold remedies to achieve a positive psychoactive effect appears to be on the increase. Many contain alcohol. People who drink these preparations to get intoxicated are running high risks of serious and often permanent damage to their liver and kidneys. In fact, the renal (kidney) failure in the 23-year-old woman was mainly due to the 6,000 mg of paracetamol, an ingredient that is relatively safe in recommended doses. Because she drank habitually she was more prone to the liver toxicity associated with high doses of this painkiller.

Clear Lungs and a Dry Nose

Many OTC cold remedies contain substances that manufacturers claim are *expectorants*. Expectorants loosen the mucus in the lungs that collects during a common cold or flu. Expectoration is a cough that brings up mucus (also called phlegm or sputum) and is beneficial because the coughed-up material contains particles of the infecting virus. According to an FDA advisory panel, evidence that available OTC expectorants are genuinely effective is quite limited. The most widely used expectorant is guaifenesin (glyceryl guaiacolate). Other drugs that have been used as expectorants include ammonium chloride, terpin hydrate, iodides of calcium, camphor, menthol, ipecac syrup and fluid extract,

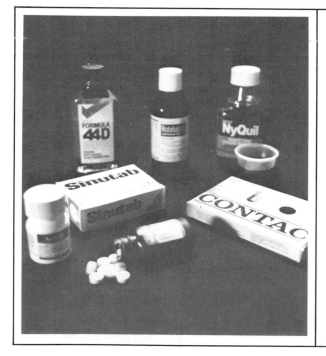

Doctors often say that a cold will last a week if medicine is given, and seven days if left alone. Although some of the popular cold medications—most of which contain alcohol—relieve cold symptoms, none will cure the cold.

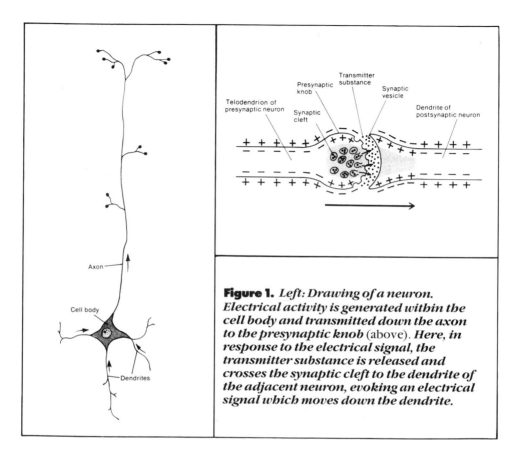

Figure 1. *Left: Drawing of a neuron. Electrical activity is generated within the cell body and transmitted down the axon to the presynaptic knob* (above). *Here, in response to the electrical signal, the transmitter substance is released and crosses the synaptic cleft to the dendrite of the adjacent neuron, evoking an electrical signal which moves down the dendrite.*

turpentine oil and chloroform. Most people are not aware that these drugs may not be effective, and that some, such as chloroform, ipecac fluid extract and turpentine oil, are potentially dangerous.

The term *anticholinergic* is derived from the word acetylcholine (ACh). ACh is one of the chemical substances, or *neurotransmitters,* that acts as a messenger between neurons in the central nervous system. Neurons are specialized cells that have long wire-like protrusions called *axons* at one end. A bundle of axons constitutes a nerve. These axons communicate with other neuronal cell bodies, but their contact is not physical. There is a small space, called a *synaptic gap,* between the end of one axon and the cell body of the next neuron. When an electrical message reaches the end of the axon, the message has to cross this synapse, and this is accomplished by neurotransmitters such as ACh.

The ACh molecule—a "translation" of the electrical charges—travels across the synaptic gap to specialized plug-ins called *receptor sites*. These are located on the numerous hair-like structures, called *dendrites*, which protrude from the cell body of the next neuron. Once a sufficient quantity of ACh molecules becomes attached to these receptor sites, a new electrical charge is set up that travels along the axon of that neuron to the next neuron, and so on.

Anticholinergic drugs alter the normal communication between neurons by binding to the receptor sites. Therefore, when ACh arrives it cannot deliver its message because the receptor sites are already full and transmitted ACh messages are never received. The result is that several bodily organs

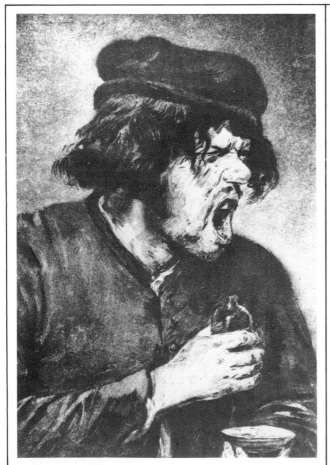

"Bitter Medicine", a painting by Flemish artist Adrian Brouwer (1606-1638). It was once widely believed that the worse a medicine tasted, the better it was for the patient. Today's pharmaceutical companies, however, work hard to make their products easy to take—and to sell.

and structures—including parts of the brain, lungs, eyes, skeletal muscles, digestive system smooth muscles and various other tissues—receive scrambled messages. Because of this binding property, anticholinergics can cause insomnia, agitation, disorientation, increased heart rate, blurred vision, constipation, hallucinations and altered judgment.

Though a runny nose may be somewhat annoying, anticholinergic drugs should not be used to alleviate it. In fact, postnasal drip is beneficial. Just as coughing clears the lungs, mucus running from the nose helps to rid the body of foreign substances.

The OTC anticholinergic drugs which have properties that dry up a runny nose are derived from the belladonna plant, also called deadly nightshade. Some of these drugs are atropine, scopolamine and hyoscyamine. Belladonna alkaloids are found in older packages of cold remedies such as

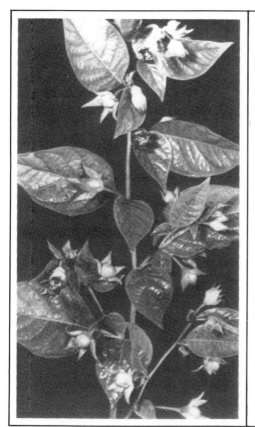

A member of the potato family, belladonna ("beautiful lady" in Italian), or the deadly nightshade, has been used since ancient times for cosmetic and medical purposes. Because the Romans considered enlarged eyes a sign of beauty, they used the drug, which causes pupil dilation, to enhance their appearance. When abused, belladonna can cause fatal reactions. Today atropine, which diminishes secretions and relieves spasms and pain, is extracted from belladonna and added to such medications as sleeping pills, anaesthetics, anti-ulcer treatments, and OTC cold remedies.

Contac Capsules. At recommended dose levels these drugs can have side effects. Drying up the air passages leaves the surfaces without protection, which can easily result in a dry, irritating, unproductive cough. Fatigue and/or excitation are common side effects due to the drug's neurological action. Dry mouth and thirst, constipation, a quickening of the heart, mental confusion and blurred vision may occur in sensitive individuals.

In higher-than-recommended doses, anticholinergic drugs are quite toxic and can induce hallucinations, altered moods and impairment of judgment. In addition, anticholinergics aggravate glaucoma (an eye disease characterized by an increase in pressure within the eye which ultimately leads to blindness). At doses considered safe for OTC drugs anticholinergics are not very effective in reducing excessive nasal discharge or watering eyes.

In the early 1980s the American Food and Drugs Administration prohibited the sale of any cold remedies that contain anticholinergics. Many consumers, however, still have cold medications that are months or even years old and contain anticholinergics. Though these drugs are no longer sold over the counter, there is no way to stop people from using these potentially dangerous substances.

To Clear the Airways

Bronchodilators, which act by dilating the bronchi of the lungs, clear the air passages and aid breathing. They are also intended to aid in expectoration and decongestion. The main category of OTC bronchodilator drugs are the ephedrine-related substances pseudoephedrine hydrochloride (HCl) and ephedrine sulphate, which have similar effects. Both drugs may cause hypertension (high blood pressure), restlessness, agitation and, with high doses, psychotic behaviour. Though bronchodilators are essential in the treatment of asthma, they are not recommended for the treatment of colds because of their potentially dangerous side effects.

Asthma Remedies

During an asthma attack a person has difficulty breathing. The remedies for asthma are drugs related to the adrenal gland hormone epinephrine, also known as adrenaline, and include ephedrine, isoproterenol (or isoprenaline) and metaproterenol. While the drugs are quite effective initially, *tolerance* develops, often rapidly. This means that to obtain relief from breathing difficulties, more and more of the drug is required. And with the increase in dosage come side effects, such as nervousness and rapid heartbeat.

Metaproterenol became available as an OTC asthma remedy in the United States in March 1983. It was marketed under the name Alupent and heavily advertised on television as a "prescription-strength" product, which, in fact, it was. Soon after metaproterenol appeared as a nonprescription drug, it became apparent that the use of this product could be fatal. At recommended doses metaproterenol is an effective and essentially safe product. However, because of the user's rapid development of tolerance, asthma sufferers are likely to abuse the drug.

Considering the extreme discomfort asthma patients may experience during an attack and the immediate relief

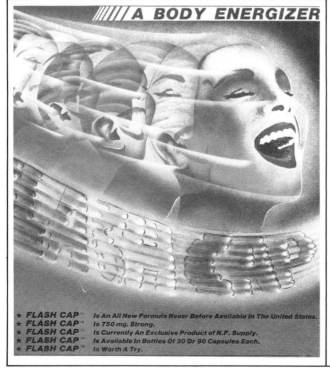

///// A BODY ENERGIZER

★ FLASH CAP™ Is An All New Formula Never Before Available In The United States.
★ FLASH CAP™ Is 750 mg. Strong.
★ FLASH CAP™ Is Currently An Exclusive Product of N.F. Supply.
★ FLASH CAP™ Is Available In Bottles Of 30 Or 90 Capsules Each.
★ FLASH CAP™ Is Worth A Try.

Among the "mental alertness aids" offered in a magazine advertisement is ephedrine, which is often used to relieve symptoms of asthma. This OTC drug produces such side effects as trembling, insomnia and rapid heartbeat.

offered by repeated inhalation of metaproterenol, that this drug is abused is not surprising. Unfortunately, when a person continuously inhales this drug the recommended doses are exceeded and progressive obstruction of the airways may be masked. This condition can lead to total respiratory collapse and even death. Because of its high abuse potential and the associated risks, metaproterenol is no longer available as an OTC drug.

Theophylline, formerly an antiasthmatic prescription drug, is now an OTC product in some countries. It is not, however, marketed as a single ingredient, but rather in combination with other substances. The doses of theophylline provided in the OTC product may not be sufficient to produce relief from an asthma attack, and therefore there is potential for abuse. The drugs with which theophylline is combined can be dangerous at the levels that are high enough to contain sufficient amounts of theophylline to have a therapeutic effect. Some preparations in addition to containing theophylline, also contain various combinations of

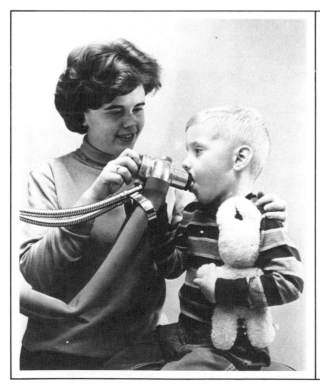

A hospital technician uses a spirometer to test the lung capacity of a five-year-old who has suffered from asthma since he was six months old. Bronchodilators metaproterenol and theophylline were both OTC drugs used to treat asthmatics. Though they can be dangerous and have a potential for abuse, only metaproterenol is no longer available as a nonprescription drug.

ephedrine, guaifenesin, and pyrilamine maleate or pheno-barbital (a barbiturate—a category of drugs that depress the central nervous system and have dangerous side effects if taken in excess). Theophylline also has a narrow safety margin. Ingesting a quantity just slightly above the recommended dosage can be dangerous. Thus there is a very delicate balance between doses that are ineffectual and those that are hazardous. Drugs orginally intended as safe medications can ultimately become a threat to health.

Antihistamines

Histamine is a chemical that is found in all body tissues, including the brain and the rest of the nervous system. In the central nervous system (CNS) histamine acts as a neuro-transmitter, while outside the nervous system histamine plays an important part in inflammation and allergic reactions.

When a tissue is infected, damaged or disturbed in any way, histamine is released from the cells in and around the affected area. Histamine's action on the surrounding capillar-ies allows larger amounts of fluid, protein, white blood cells and *macrophages* (specialized cells that get rid of unwanted foreign substances and dead tissue) to pass from the capil-laries and initiate the healing process. This sudden accumu-lation of substances is what is known as inflammation. Thus histamine and the associated inflammation play a very im-portant role in the process by which the body prevents the spread of infection to neighbouring tissues.

There are many people whose bodies are extremely sensitive to insect bites, pollen and even dust. Their inflam-matory defence mechanism is activated in response to any of these events. To most people a mosquito bite is only a minor irritation that results in a small welt. In allergic indi-viduals (i.e., people with a highly sensitive system) the same bite may cause severe inflammation all over the body. If a nonallergic person enters a room where the pollen count has been artificially elevated to ten times the 'highest con-centration possible out in the open air, even he or she may sneeze, get congested and have a runny nose and watery, itchy, red eyes. This is the body's way of getting rid of any pollen that has already invaded his or her body, and of preventing more of the pollen from entering his or her lungs and eyes. In allergic individuals much lower concentrations of pollen induce the same allergic reaction.

An antihistamine is a drug that inhibits the action of histamine and thus reduces or eliminates the allergic response. Therefore, the annoying red eyes, sneezing and runny nose are relieved. Most antihistamines are sedating and thus cause fatigue; they should be used cautiously if one is driving a car or operating any potentially dangerous

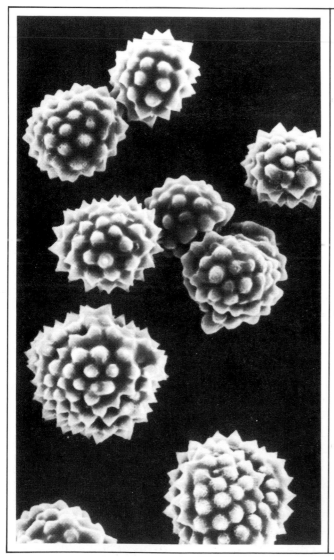

Pollen, released into the air by plants during their reproductive phase, appears to the naked eye as fine dust. However, when magnified 1,100 times, it becomes evident that pollen is actually composed of countless microspores. In those individuals who are highly sensitive, these jagged particles cause allergic reactions, characterized by sneezing, congestion, runny nose and watery, itchy eyes.

machinery. OTC antihistamines that are widely used alone or in combination include diphenhydramine (Benylin), doxylamine pyrilamine, chlorpheniramine (Piriton) and brompheniramine.

Nasal Decongestants

One of the most bothersome symptoms of a cold or flu is a congested, or stuffed, nose. To help get rid of this symptom the consumer can take a topical drug (inhalants, sprays or drops) or an oral decongestant (pills or syrups). The disadvantages of pills and syrups is that they take much longer to act than inhalants, sprays and drops, and they can also have many undesirable effects on the body. For example, if used topically (ingested through the nose) as recommended, ephedrine sulphate, phenylpropanolamine (PPA) and phenylephrine, three drugs used in nasal decongestants, produce the desired localized decongestant effect and do not affect the rest of the body.

All three of these drugs, however, affect the *catecholamines*, neurotransmitters such as epinephrine (adrenaline) and dopamine. Therefore, if they are taken orally in high doses they can affect neurons and nerves throughout the whole body and cause hypertension,

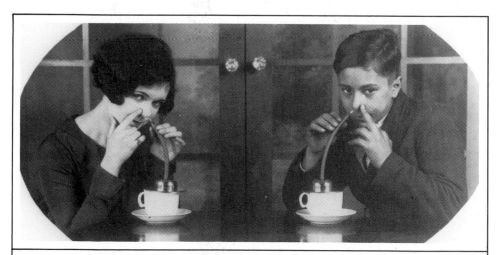

In 1925 a news story announced the discovery of "a new way to cure colds"— a "gas-generating inhaler" inserted into a cup of tea.

restlessness, agitation, sleeplessness, or even heart problems.

Topical nasal decongestants, if used for more than two or three days in a row, may cause *rebound congestion*. This has occurred when, after discontinuing drug use, the congestion actually becomes much worse than it was initially. The temptation is to resort again to the use of an inhalant to get rid of the congestion. This cycle can cause addiction to the inhalant, spray or nose drops. The only solution is to stop using the inhalant altogether. When given the chance, the body can expel the irritant that is causing this symptom, and within a few weeks the congestion will disappear.

Cough Medicines

Antitussives are substances that act to inhibit an uncontrollable, dry or unproductive cough. (The word "tussive" means related to, of the nature of, or pertaining to, a cough.) A number of medications are available, and they include codeine, dextromethorphan, diphenhydramine hydrochloride (an antihistamine), various "combination" syrups, topical products (such as menthol-containing lozenges), and chest rubs, which are often composed of half a dozen different oils and extracts.

The only truly effective cough suppressants are codeine and dextromethorphan. Codeine is one of the weakest narcotics (i.e., an opium derivative), which, apart from inhibiting the cough centre in the brain, relieves pain and produces euphoria. Its inclusion in a number of cough remedies is, however, primarily due to its cough-suppressant effects. In fact, the amount of codeine contained in the recommended doses of cough remedies is not sufficient to produce pain-relieving effects.

Codeine's potential for abuse, however, is comparatively high. Codeine-containing products may be abused in an attempt to reduce the coughing and pain due to colds, or in order to achieve the drug's euphoric effects. And excessively high doses and/or doses ingested too frequently can produce a condition of drug dependence. The liquid cold/cough formulas, which usually contain alcohol, are the forms of codeine most likely to be abused. Initially the person may be seeking the euphoric effects of either the codeine or the alcohol, but after repeated use of the combination he or she may become addicted to one or both of them. Since it is one of the weakest of the opium derived analgesics, codeine has fewer and less severe side effects.

Dextromethorphan, on the other hand, is a safe non-narcotic drug that suppresses coughing and is contained in most cough medicines. If too much is ingested, however, it will slow breathing. Unfortunately, dextromethorphan is usually only available in combinations that include up to four or five other ingredients. Because of this, when choosing a

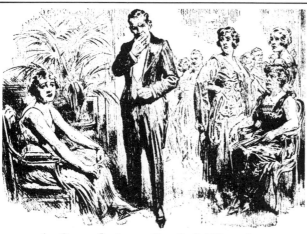

A Cough is a Social Blunder

People who know have no hesitation in avoiding the cougher. They know that he is a public menace. They know that his cough is a proof of his lack of consideration of others.

And they know that he knows it too, so S. B. Cough Drops are not a cure for colds. They are a preventive of coughing. True, they often keep a cough from developing into a sore throat or cold. And they are a protection to the public because they keep people who already have influenza, colds and other throat troubles from spreading them through unnecessary coughing. Have a box with you always.

they are not afraid of hurting his feelings.

For there is no excuse for coughing. It is just as unnecessary as any other bad habit. For it can be prevented or relieved by the simplest of precautions—the use of S. B. Cough Drops.

Pure. No Drugs. Just enough charcoal to sweeten the stomach.

One placed in the mouth at bedtime will keep the breathing passages clear.

Drop that Cough
SMITH BROTHERS of Poughkeepsie
FAMOUS SINCE 1847

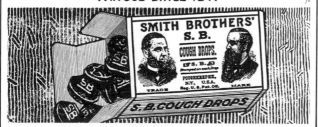

An American cough drop manufacturer, who ran this advertisement in 1919, hoped to convince "coughers" that they could avoid serious "social blunders" by using this product, which also offered "protection to the public" by preventing unnecessary coughing", for which there was "no excuse".

truly effective cough/cold medication, even the most cautious consumer is forced to ingest ineffective and potentially dangerous drugs to obtain the relief which a single, safe drug could provide.

Headache and Fever Medications

Analgesic is the technical word for pain reliever, and *antipyretics* are substances that reduce fever. Since many cough/cold remedies contain painkillers it is important to briefly consider them here.

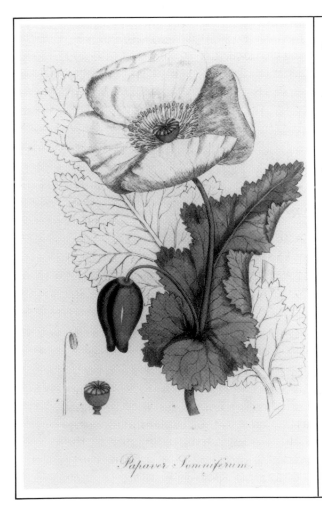

Papaver Somniferum.

The poppy **Papaver somnivorum** *produces a milky juice, which is the source of the opiates: opium, morphine, codeine, and their derivatives. Even codeine, the weakest of these drugs, has a very high potential for abuse.*

The two main analgesics and antipyretics contained in OTC cold products are acetylsalicylic acid (aspirin) and paracetamol. These two products are virtually the only analgesic/anti-inflammatory agents marketed as cold symptom relievers. Because a population has not yet been identified that is allergic to it, and because it does not irritate the stomach lining and cause bleeding (as aspirin may do), paracetamol is presently by far the favoured ingredient. However, unlike paracetamol, aspirin reduces inflammation.

A high dose of paracetamol can cause dangerous hepatotoxic (liver-damaging) effects. A common sequence of seemingly harmless events may lead to this condition. When a person consumes a product such as Rinurel he or she may not realize that it contains the analgesic paracetamol, and so in addition he or she will take a few aspirins for pain, sometimes even chasing the aspirin with alcohol. Alcohol and aspirin are both stomach irritants, and the ingested combination can make the stomach lining painfully, even dangerously, irritated. The situation and others similar to it could be avoided if the drug user read *all* the ingredients in OTC drugs and considered the effects of each one before ingesting a combination that has the potential of being hazardous and even life-threatening.

Combination Cold Remedies

Of all the OTC medications available on the market, single-ingredient cold remedies constitute only a minor portion. Today the market is flooded with combination products that contain up to five different ingredients. This "shotgun" approach for treating a cold, which would probably clear up on its own within four days, is unwarranted and potentially dangerous.

There are many reasons why this type of approach to treatment is unwarranted. Firstly, a person may not be suffering from all the symptoms—headache, sneezing, coughing, congested lungs and a stuffed up nose—at the same time. Even if a person did have all these symptoms simultaneously, the possibility is remote that each drug contained in the medication exists in the correct dosage for the successful treatment of each of these symptoms. Because of this, he or she is likely to take additional doses just to get rid of the most

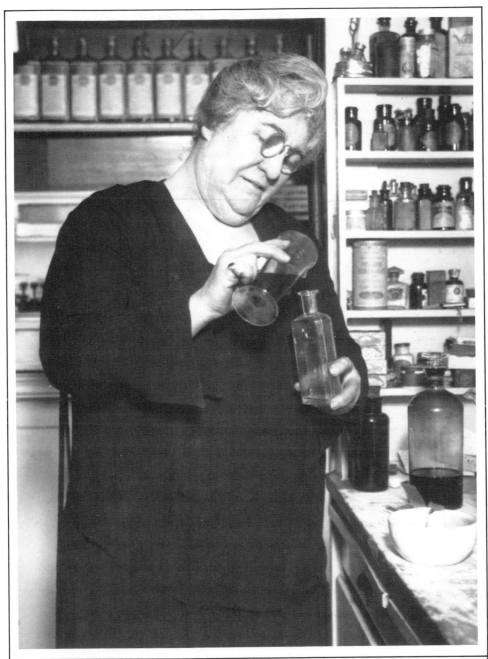

Minnie Belle McAvoy, America's first licensed female pharmacist, mixes a prescription in her Manhattan drugstore in 1924. Before federal laws were tightened, "medicine" was often dispensed by unlicensed individuals.

bothersome symptom. Meanwhile, the person receives an overdose of the other ingredients. Flu symptoms are slightly different each time they occur. Sometimes the symptoms include a sinus headache and nasal congestion; sometimes a cough, a congested chest and a mild fever; and other times just a runny nose and sneezing. Each symptom—and only if it is really unbearable—should and can be treated separately.

By using compound remedies to relieve one or two bothersome symptoms, people are taking excessive doses of too many drugs. If a person habitually does this each time he or she gets the flu, serious health problems may occur.

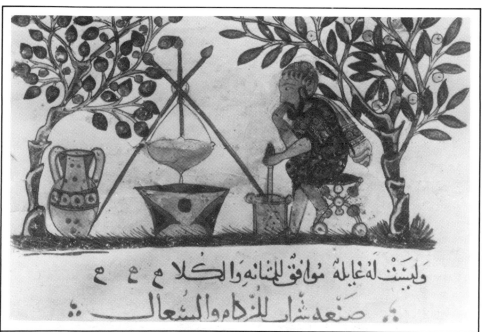

An Arabian chemist distils medicinal wine for use as a cough suppressant. The illustration is from a book about botanical medicine by Pedanius Dioscorides, a 1st-century Greek physician whose work remained the authority on this subject for 1,500 years.

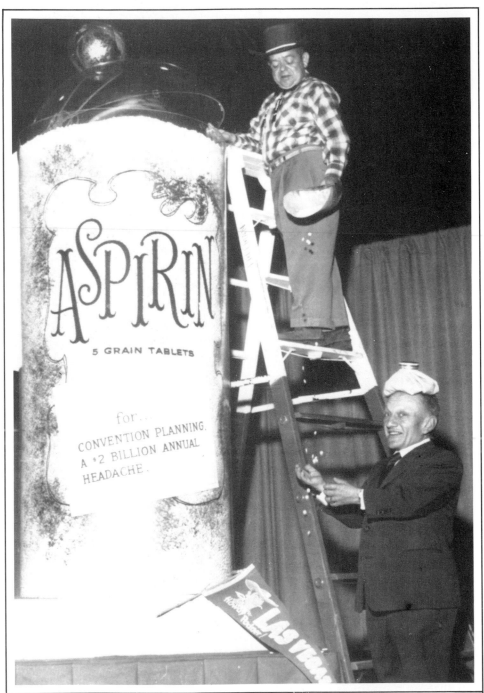

The two million aspirin tablets in this giant jar—a promotional exhibit at a Las Vegas exhibition—represent less than one-third of the aspirin consumed by Americans every hour of every day.

CHAPTER 3

PAIN RELIEF

Pain is a signal that something is wrong. Without pain it would be difficult, if not impossible, to live. For example, without pain a person would not know when to remove his or her hand from a hot radiator and would thus suffer severe burns. There are many types of pain, such as headaches, muscle aches and toothaches, all of which can be quite annoying. For many people these aches and pains are daily experiences.

Event though these pains are symptoms of some problem that needs correcting, it often seems simpler to eliminate the symptoms rather than combat the direct cause, which might in fact be serious. Because of the simplicity of this treatment and its ready availability, and because of the undeniable discomfort caused by the pain, more people purchase OTC painkillers than any other types of products.

Among OTC painkillers, aspirin and paracetamol, best known in the form of Panadol, are the most popular. Other OTC pain relievers include salicylate, salicylamide, and salsalate, which are all closely related to aspirin. These will not be discussed at any length, since they are less potent representatives of the family of *salicylates* (see Figure 2), and are, therefore, used much less frequently. Ibuprofen, a potent analgesic from a different chemical group, has joined the ranks of OTC products in the United States. It has been a prescription product, for many years, so that much is now known about its safety and efficacy.

Aspirin

In 1899, when Felix Hoffmann, a chemist at the Bayer

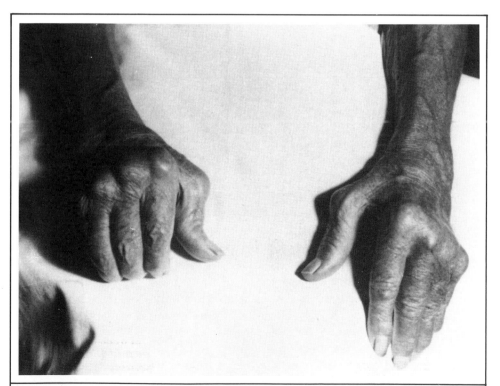

The hands of an arthritis sufferer give evidence of the crippling effects of this disease, which torments millions. Aspirin provides some relief from the pain and swelling produced by arthritis.

Company, discovered a low-cost method of synthesis for acetylsalicylic acid, better known as aspirin, he started a veritable revolution in the OTC industry. Aspirin (acetylsalicylic acid, or ASA) is a member of a group of compounds called *salicylates* (see Figure 2). Unlike the narcotic analgesics, which alter the perception of pain by acting on the central nervous system, aspirin acts locally at the source of the pain. The reduction of pain and inflammation is accomplished by vasodilation (dilation of blood vessels) and by a decrease in the production of *prostaglandins*, chemicals in the body that, along with histamines, are released during inflammation. When a fever is present, aspirin reduces body temperature by causing superficial (surface) blood vessels to dilate. But while this enables the body to dissipate more heat, it does not reduce actual heat production. In addition, research has shown that a fever is part of the body's mechanism to fight disease; therefore, reducing a fever actually slows down the healing process.

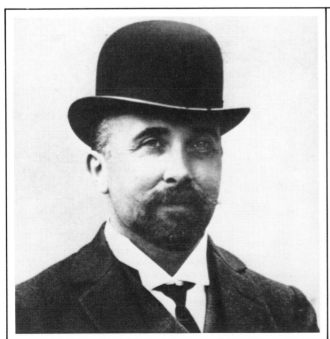

German Chemist Felix Hoffmann (1868-1946) paved the way for the commercial production of aspirin, which had first been synthesized in the mid-1800s. He became interested in the drug when he discovered that it gave his father relief from arthritis pain.

The major problem with aspirin is that it irritates the stomach lining, sometimes to the point of bleeding, and can lead to gastric and peptic ulcers. Prolonged use of aspirin may also interfere with the clotting of blood after an injury. To reduce aspirin's stomach-irritant properties, antacids have been included in a number of aspirin formulations. However, studies have repeatedly shown that with regards to stomach irritation, these products offer no significant advantage over plain aspirin taken with a glass of water.

People suffering from arthritis are highly prone to take near toxic doses of aspirin. Arthritis is characterized by inflamed joints which, when moved or put under stress, cause pain. Since aspirin reduces inflammation and pain, it is the drug most suggested for treatment of arthritis. Although the suggested adult dose is two 325-mg tablets four times a day, many sufferers will take much higher levels to reduce the inflammation and the pain. This amount of aspirin can cause salicylate toxicity, symptoms of which include dizziness, ringing in the ears, gastrointestinal problems, mental confusion and bleeding. Clearly, these undesirable effects should be avoided as much as possible.

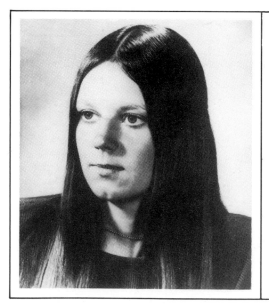

In 1975, 21-year-old Karen Anne Quinlan became the centre of a highly publicized "right-to-die" case when her parents sought to discontinue life supports after she went into a coma. Tests showed that she had consumed a small amount of alcohol along with aspirin and, possibly, Valium. Even after the case was won and the life-support system was disconnected, she remained alive, unconscious until her death ten years later.

Alka-Seltzer is widely advertised for the relief of an upset stomach. However, a recommended dose contains appreciable levels of salicylate. Therefore, if someone who is already taking high doses of aspirin—ingests Alka-Seltzer, he or she is unknowlingly exposing him- or herself to a potential hazard. This combination of medications could result in a toxic salicylate level.

Believe it or not, some people take aspirin just to get high. Ten years ago there were stories that claimed that mixing aspirin with Coca-Cola was guaranteed to give you a "buzz". But by far the most common form of abuse is associated with taking far too much aspirin. This is usually done based on the incorrect assumption that if a small dose makes you feel better, then a larger one should make you

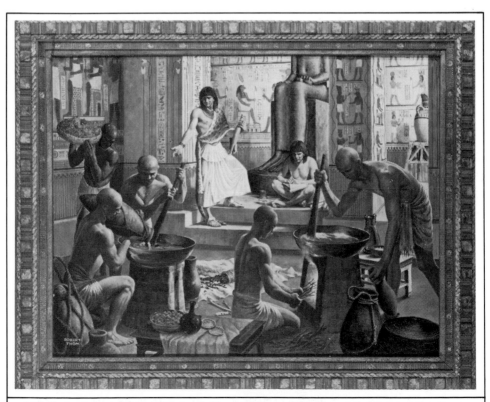

A 20-th century artist's interpretation of Days of the Papyrus Ebers, *a book first published in 1500 B.C., shows an Egyptian doctor directing the preparation of medical potions. The book mentioned seven hundred drugs.*

feel great. This faulty reasoning has led to serious and even fatal overdoses. And yet, people obviously know that a high dose of aspirin can cause death. In the 1980s, aspirin, after barbiturates, is the drug of choice in suicide attempts.

Paracetamol

Paracetamol (N-acetylpara-aminophenol, or APAP) is as potent an analgesic and antipyretic as aspirin, but it has no effect on inflammation. As Figure 2 illustrates, their chemical structures are also very similar. Paracetamol has advantages over aspirin in that it does not necessarily irritate the gastro-intestinal tract or other mucous membranes, and in recommended doses its side effects are negligible. Although paracetamol is not anti-inflammatory, it is useful in alleviating arthritic pain.

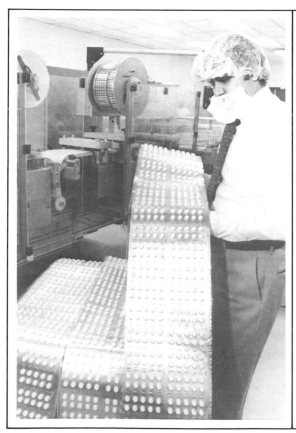

A technician inspects blister-pack strips of aspirin-free tablets. The pills contain paracetamol, an aspirin substitute that is increasingly used to combat arthritis pain.

Figure 2. *The chemical structure of four painkillers. All have a central benzene ring to which are attached additional atoms, which determine each one's particular characteristics. Note the similarities between aspirin and salicylate and between acetophenetidin and paracetamol.*

SOURCE: Adapted from *Review of Medical Pharmacology.* F. H. Myers, E. Jawetz and A. Goldfien (Eds.), Los Altos: Lange, 1978.

Aspirin and Paracetamol Compared

The pharmaceutical industry has been spending millions of dollars in advertising campaigns in the aspirin-versus-paracetamol controversy. Many people who are allergic to aspirin or are predisposed to its stomach-irritating properties have been made aware of the alternative. However, many of the pharmaceutical companies have marketed both aspirin and paracetamol and given them similar names. This practice has made the process of acquiring accurate information and making intelligent decisions that much more complicated.

The major disadvantage of paracetamol use is its potential for overdose toxicity. Though at recommended doses and frequency it poses no dangers, high doses can cause severe and sometimes fatal liver damage. On the other hand, even extremely high doses of aspirin, which can cause hallucinations, convulsions and coma, are not likely to be fatal if treated in time. Long-term use of paracetamol at recommended doses has not yet been shown to be hazardous —hepatotoxicity usually only develops from massive overdoses. Long-term aspirin use, however, can result in gastrointestinal disorders. On the other hand, aspirin has the advantage over paracetamol of being able to reduce inflammation as well as pain; paracetamol only relieves the pain.

Recent evidence suggests that aspirin may have beneficial effects in addition to its pain-relieving and anti-inflammatory effects. Regular use of aspirin seems to prevent the development of senile cataracts and the deterioration of the eye lens. It is also thought to be effective in the treatment of myocardial infarction (i.e., heart muscle degeneration due to inadequate blood flow), and in reducing the incidence of reinfarction. It has also been used successfully in alleviating transient ischaemic attacks (i.e., decreased blood supply to localized tissues). In infarction and ischaemia treatment, for some as yet unknown reason, men seem to benefit more than women.

Paracetamol has only been on the market for thirty years (whereas the family of salicylates was first identified in 1829, and its most prominent member, aspirin, was isolated seventy years later). Because of its recent emergence, not all of paracetamol's positive and negative effects have been determined.

Every year, a substantial number of children accidentally

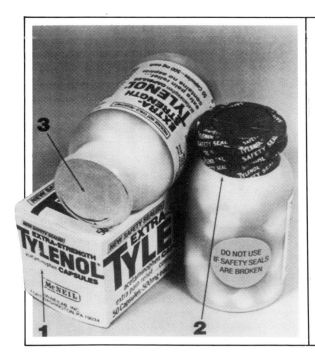

In 1982 Tylenol, the most popular OTC form of paracetamol in the United States, was temporarily withdrawn from the market after several of its users had mysteriously died. They were discovered to have been poisoned by cyanide, which had been inserted into Tylenol packages after they had been placed on store shelves. Later that same year the drug was reintroduced in triple-sealed packages.

overdose on aspirin or paracetamol, sometimes with fatal results. Analgesics manufactured for children are usually sugar-coated, or even "chewable", like sweets. Many youngsters, unaware that the pills are medicine, do in fact eat them as if they were sweets.

The aspirin/paracetamol controversy has had the beneficial effect of bringing the possible health hazards of aspirin use to everyone's attention. Since the most common problem is stomach irritation, the drug manufacturers have provided the consumer with a wide choice of coated pills and capsules. Unfortunately, though coated pills may offer some protection for the mucosal lining of the mouth and

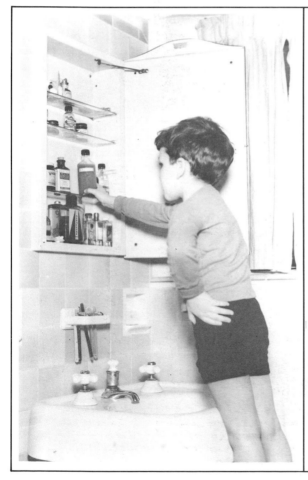

Because children are naturally both curious about and imitative of their parents, an unlocked medicine cabinet containing drugs—either prescription or OTC—is an open invitation to tragedy.

oesophageal tube, they do not protect the stomach. Despite warnings, many people still take regular, uncoated aspirin tablets without any liquid. This practice has an effect on the mouth and oesophageal lining similar to drinking slightly diluted hydrochloric acid. Aspirin is called acetylsalicylic *acid* because it *is* an acid, and a pretty strong one at that. Therefore, whether coated or not, aspirin should always be ingested with water or milk which dilutes it, but not with alcohol, which by itself can damage the stomach lining.

Since aspirin- and paracetamol-containing products are the medications that are by far the most widely advertised and "prescribed" by both the media and physicians, and because these products can successfully treat the majority of aches and pains, they are often taken indiscriminately. To ensure that they are equipped to deal with minor ailments at all times, many households stock aspirin-and/or paracetamol-containing remedies. In theory there is nothing wrong with having these medicines on hand. One just has to exercise self-control and use them wisely. Firstly, their accessibility poses a danger for children, who may unknowingly and indiscriminately take them as sweets. Secondly, even responsible adults, when they are not feeling well are likely to take anything readily available and not necessarily what is therapeutic.

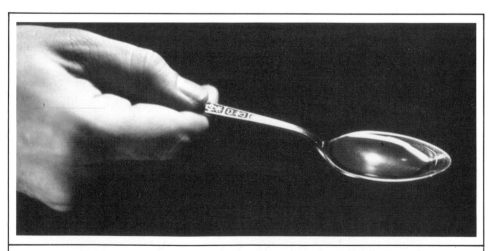

The size of a recommended dose is determined from careful scientific studies. "One spoonful" means just that; two may be dangerous.

This practice can lead to psychological as well as to physical dependence. A high percentage of liquid OTC cough and cold remedies contain up to 600 mg of paracetamol per spoonful, the common recommended dose. But quite frequently the recommended spoonful turns out to be a couple of "slurps" out of the bottle, a few times a day. More or less naively, many individuals do this and thus invite serious health problems.

Phenacetin

Phenacetin is very closely related to paracetamol, but despite this close chemical relationship phenacetin has been proven to be very dangerous. It has been identified as a carcinogen, and its prolonged use has been strongly correlated with a high incidence of kidney disease and anaemia. In addition to its analgesic effect it can also cause drowsiness and mild euphoria.

Because of its sedative and euphoric effects and its reputation as an anxiety reliever, phenacetin has a high abuse potential. This and other dangers were clearly recognized in the mid-1970s, but it was not until early in the 1980s that the decision was made to remove it from the market. Phenacetin is mentioned here because it is possible that many households still have products which contain it. Because of their dangerous side effects, products containing phenacetin should be thrown away.

Codeine

When found in OTC products, codeine is marketed both as a cough suppressant and as an analgesic. When an antitussive product is used in recommended doses, and only for its intended purpose, the analgesic properties are not very strong. When used as an analgesic, however, the dosage is some three to six times higher. Codeine-containing OTC products may cause sedation. The previously mentioned problem of overdosing on the other ingredients of a combination product is also of major concern here. But the greatest hazard that results from using codeine for its pain-relieving effects is the relatively high addiction potential.

Pain Reliever Boosters

Caffeine and many of the antihistamines are often added to painkillers to enhance their effects. When used for this purpose these other drugs are called adjuvants. Since practically no evidence exists of the effectiveness of antihistamines in this role, they will not be included in this discussion. The evidence that caffeine enhances the pain-relieving effect of analgesics (e.g., aspirin and paracetamol), though not conclusive, is much stronger than it is for antihistamines.

Caffeine (trimethylxanthine) is found in coffee, tea, Coca Cola, Pepsi, and chocolate-containing foods. It has mild CNS-stimulating properties, and in the United States is often sold over the counter in pill form alone (i.e., No Doz) or in combination with PPA or ephedrine, and advertised as either a stimulant or diet aid. Caffeine appears to exert its CNS-

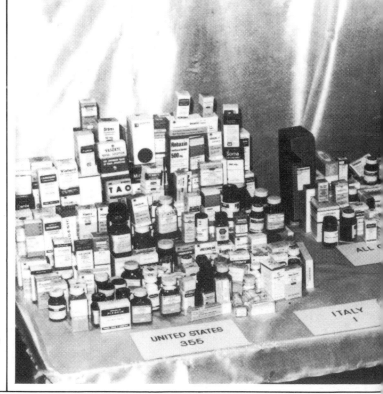

A comparison of medicines developed between 1941 and 1964 by the world's pharmaceutical companies illustrates how the United States is by far the world's leading drug-producing nation.

stimulating effects by blocking *adenosine* receptors. Adenosine is another chemical thought to be a neurotransmitter.

As an ingredient in painkillers caffeine is supposed to enhance the overall analgesic effect. However, some experts claim that it is useless and, in fact, a hazard. An editorial in the *Journal of the American Medical Association* maintained that most previous studies investigating caffeine's enhancement of aspirin or paracetamol used too low a dose of caffeine, i.e., 32 mg–64 mg. One study found that 1.4 times as much aspirin or paracetamol is required to equal the analgesic effect of a combination of a given amount of either drug and 65 mg of caffeine. Because the 65 mg of caffeine was contained in each tablet of painkiller, a normal dose of two or three tablets would contain 130 mg or 195 mg of caffeine, equivalent to 1½ to 2½ cups of coffee (see Table 3).

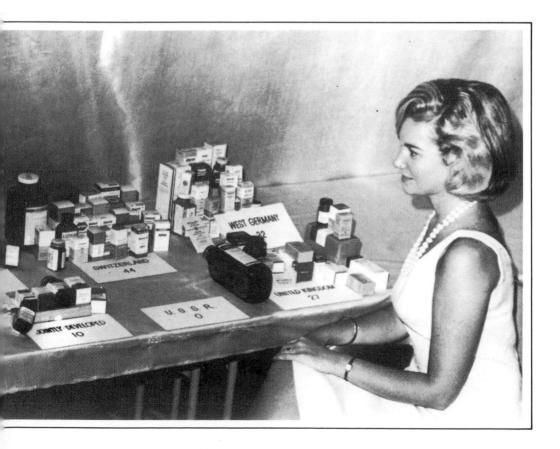

Although it is true that 200 mg of caffeine can usually be tolerated by most people, problems can arise.

People often take up a dozen painkillers in a day to subdue severe cold symptoms, headaches or toothaches. This means that they may be ingesting up to 780 mg of caffeine. Combined with other sources of caffeine, their total daily caffeine intake may be more than 1,000 mg. To get this much caffeine one would have to drink seven cups of strongly brewed coffee.

Caffeine, like so many other drugs, can cause physical dependence. For example, someone who habitually drinks three to six cups of coffee each day during the work week, but only one or two cups at weekends may experience "migraines", an uncomfortable withdrawal symptom. The brain's adenosine receptors, accustomed to their daily "caffeine fix", respond to the decrease of caffeine and a headache results. Most people are not aware that just drinking their usual amount of coffee would alleviate the discomfort, and instead they take painkillers. In fact, they will probably discover that such caffeine-containing painkillers as Excedrin or Anacin provide the most relief for them.

Maintaining such high levels of caffeine is not healthy (see Chapter 4), and alleviating weekend caffeine-withdrawal headaches with caffeine-containing remedies perpetuates the coffee/caffeine addiction. The clever and economical way out of this vicious cycle is to cut down on coffee consumption.

Combination Products

Products with two or more active ingredients seem to appeal to the general public. This is as true for cold remedies as it is for painkillers. At first glance, combining aspirin, paracetamol and caffeine in order to enhance the overall analgesic effect does not seem unreasonable. And there are an appreciable number of products on the market that contain two or more analgesics in addition to other active ingredients.

When only pain is the issue, a "shotgun" approach makes some sense. Headaches, toothaches, backaches and cramps obviously have different causes, but the symptom is the same—pain. However, the subjective experience of the pain might be different. Headaches alone can vary in intensity, specific location, duration and quality (i.e., dull, throbbing, sharp or piercing). Because of the wide range of sensations and because no product claims to relieve a specific type of pain, people often conclude that a product containing two or three different painkillers is much more likely to alleviate the type of pain from which they are suffering.

Though there have been numerous studies, none has concluded that combination products are significantly more effective in reducing pain than either paracetamol or aspirin alone. Therefore, there is no reason to risk the combined side effects of these products.

Menstrual Pain

Prior to a woman's menstrual period it is not uncommon for her to suffer from what is called *premenstrual syndrome*. This condition is characterized by fluid retention, or bloating, sensitive or painful breasts and irritability. And during actual menstrual bleeding uterine contractions may cause severe cramps and pain. To eliminate these symptoms many women turn to various products specifically marketed to treat

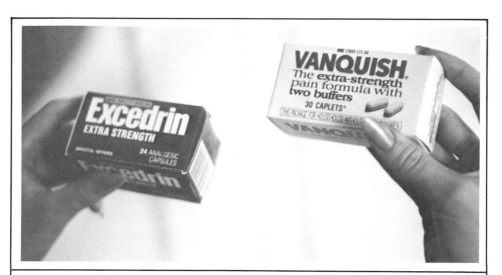

Anxious to relieve symptoms as quickly as possible, many drug users ingest combination products and risk the combined side effects. There is no solid evidence that such combinations increase effectiveness.

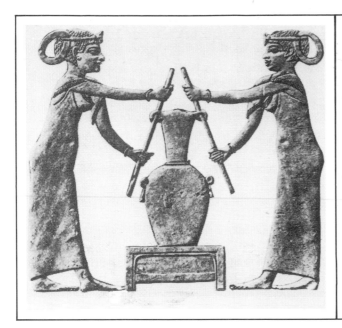

Female apothecaries prepare herbal medicine in ancient Egypt. In treating "women's complaints" over the centuries, druggists have used potions containing many varieties of herbs, belladonna, and other potent substances. The major ingredient of "Lydia Pinkham's Organic Compound", a popular American medicine for women in the early 1900s, was cocaine.

premenstrual syndrome. However, none of the ingredients, other than the painkillers, have been proved to be effective in treating premenstrual syndrome.

In fact, the best way to reduce fluid buildup is to decrease salt intake for a week or so before menstruation. If this does not help, professional medical care should be sought. Ibuprofen has proved to be more effective in relieving menstrual cramps than aspirin or paracetamol, though there have been reports of fluid retention associated with high doses.

CHAPTER 4

STIMULANTS AND DIET AIDS

*T*he terms "overweight" and "obese" mean different things to different people. However, it is generally accepted that being overweight or obese refers to the condition of exceeding acceptable weight standards for a given height. Although sometimes total body/water calculations or skinfold thickness are used, the most common way to determine if one's weight falls within an acceptable range is to compare it with the figures on an ideal weight table (see Table 2). Regardless of the criteria used, it is safe to say that today 20% of people weigh more than they should.

In the 1950s it was common for doctors to prescribe amphetamines (also known as "speed" or "uppers") for obesity. And frequently they were given to depressed patients, who lacked the motivation to function normally. When amphetamines were prescribed as anorectics (appetite suppressants), initially they did help the patient lose weight, but tolerance rapidly developed, necessitating higher doses of amphetamine to produce the desired effect. When increasing daily dosages were prescribed, the dieter was able to maintain the new weight, but not without paying the price.

The situation is like running high-octane racing fuel in a 1969 Volkswagen. At first the car will drive as if it were

Table 2

Ideal Weight Table								
Height	**Men's Weight**				**Women's Weight**			
	Average		Acceptable Weight Range		Average		Acceptable Weight Range	
(ft in) m	St lb	Kg	St lb	Kg	St lb	Kg	St lb	Kg
4-10 1.47					7-4	45.9	6-8 – 8-7	41.4–53.6
4-11 1.50					7-6	46.8	6-10– 8-10	42.3–54.9
5- 0 1.52					7-9	48.2	6-12– 8-13	43.2–56.3
5- 1 1.55					7-12	49.5	7-1 – 9-2	44.6–57.6
5- 2 1.57	8-11	55.4	8-0 –10-1	50.4–63.5	8-1	50.9	7-4 – 9-5	45.9–59.0
5- 3 1.60	9-1	57.2	8-3 –10-4	51.8–64.8	8-4	52.2	7-7 – 9-8	47.3–60.3
5- 4 1.63	9-4	58.5	8-6 –10-8	53.1–66.6	8-8	54.0	7-10– 9-12	48.6–62.1
5- 5 1.65	9-7	59.9	8-9 –10-12	54.5–68.4	8-11	55.4	7-13–10-2	50.0–63.9
5- 6 1.68	9-11	61.2	8-12–11.2	55.8–70.2	9-2	57.6	8-2 –10-6	51.3–65.7
5- 7 1.70	10-0	63.0	9-2 –11-7	57.6–72.5	9-6	59.4	8-6 –10-10	53.1–67.5
5- 8 1.73	10-5	65.3	9-6 –11-12	59.4–74.7	9-10	61.2	8-10–11.00	54.9–69.3
5- 9 1.75	10-9	67.1	9-10–12-2	61.2–76.5	10-0	63.0	9-0 –11-4	56.7–71.1
5-10 1.78	10-13	68.9	10-0 –12-6	63.0–78.3	10-4	64.8	9-4 –11-9	58.5–73.4
5-11 1.80	11-4	71.1	10-4 –12-11	64.8–80.6	10-8	66.6	9-8 –12-0	60.3–75.6
6- 0 1.83	11-8	72.9	10-8 –13.2	66.6–82.8	10-12	68.4	9-12–12-5	62.1–77.9
6- 1 1.85	11-12	74.7	10-12–13-7	68.4–85.1				
6- 2 1.88	12-3	77.0	11-2 –13-12	70.2–87.3				
6- 3 1.90	12-8	79.2	11-6 –14-3	72.0–89.6				
6- 4 1.93	12-13	81.5	11-10–14-8	73.8–91.8				

new, but soon troubles such as overheating of the upper cylinders (a condition aggravated by continued use of the high-octane fuel) will develop. Similarly, a person ingesting increasing doses of amphetamine will begin exhibiting psychotic-like symptoms (often indistinguishable from paranoid schizophrenia): heart palpitations, nervousness, agitation that can lead to violence, digestive problems and, as the amphetamine wears off, depression. The "speed freaks" of the late 1960s and early 1970s were living testimony to the side effects of prolonged amphetamine use.

The chances are just as high that these same side effects will occur when amphetamine is prescribed to alleviate depression or given to a person to increase the motivation to cope with his or her daily problems. Simply, the human body functions better for a little while, but then every system begins to exhibit symptoms of being overworked.

Whether amphetamines are used to combat lethargy or obesity, only short-term relief is accomplished. As past studies have shown, even patients who have every intention of using the amphetamine as prescribed find themselves taking greater and greater amounts and seeing a dozen or more doctors to obtain prescriptions for amphetamines. Many users entered the black market and sold a portion of their pills for more than they themselves had paid. The profit easily covered their own costs.

Physicians and the public finally became aware of the amphetamine-related problems, and as a result, tighter restrictions were enforced. In the 1970s there was a steady decline in the number of prescriptions for amphetamines.

Substitutes for Amphetamines

It is important to understand the effects of amphetamine, a prescription drug, for two reasons. Firstly, today people are buying OTC diet aids and stimulants for exactly the same reasons as they had previously bought amphetamines: to use them to lose weight, to feel energetic and stay awake, and to

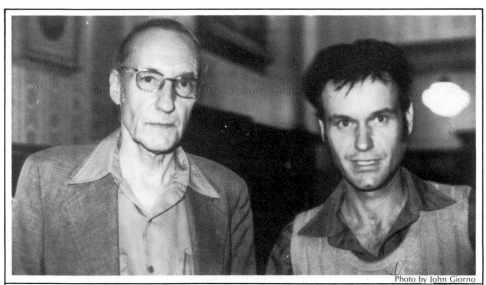

Photo by John Giorno

William Burroughs, Jr., (right) posing with his father, the writer William S. Burroughs, was greatly influenced by the Beat Generation's insatiable thirst for extreme experiences. He died at the early age of thirty-three, after a life of drug (especially amphetamine) abuse.

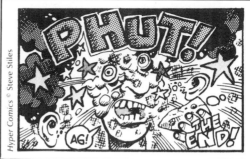

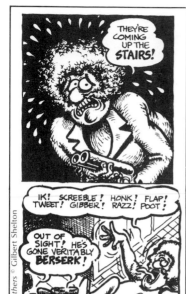

These three scenes from popular comics illustrate some of the effects of amphetamine abuse: paranoia (top, left); slurred speech and talkativeness (left); and psychosis, including hallucinations and violent behaviour.

get "high", and to sell them on the black market for a profit. Secondly, the ingredients of these OTC drugs can produce similar types of dangerous side effects.

How did this situation come about? Today doctors are very hesitant to prescribe amphetamines for any reason. Studies have shown that for the average person, the only way to keep excess pounds off is to use common sense. For most of us who lead relatively sedentary lives it would be wise to exercise more and eat less. For those who cringe at the thought of any kind of prolonged, sweaty activity, taking a pill is more tempting.

Many people would also prefer to take an "energy" pill to deal more effectively with their day-to-day problems rather than to invest greater effort in developing more productive sleeping, working and recreational habits. Pharmaceutical companies are quite aware of our weaknesses and use their knowledge to create seductive advertisements that promise easy solutions. They offer a wide variety of products, but most of them contain the same basic ingredients: caffeine, phenylpropanolamine (PPA), and ephedrine derivatives (ephedrine sulphate, ephedrine hydrochloride and pseudoephedrine). And in many ways these drugs are similar to amphetamines.

Caffeine

Caffeine is a stimulant used by people around the world. It is a major ingredient in coffee, which is why people drink it to get going in the morning and to keep them going when they get tired. The caffeine content of some common beverages is listed in Table 3. Derived from a class of drugs called *xanthines*, caffeine is a central nervous system stimulant that specifically stimulates the brain. It has been associated with anxiety, heart disease, gastrointestinal irritation and ulcers.

Stimulants and diet pills contain up to 325 mg of caffeine per tablet or capsule. This means that even if one were to abstain from all other sources of caffeine (which is often difficult, since many drinks, foods and other OTC and prescription drugs also contain caffeine), two diet pills a day would provide an amount of caffeine equivalent to about five cups of coffee. Because the potential for ingesting a large amount of caffeine is very great, the risk of suffering from the hazardous side effects increases.

Table 3

Caffeine Content in Common Beverages		
AMOUNT	BEVERAGE	CAFFEINE CONTENT (mg)
1 cup	Percolated coffee*	80–150
1 cup	Instant coffee	50–75
1 cup	Decaffeinated coffee	3–6
1 cup	Tea*	20–100
12 oz	Cola	50

*Caffeine content depends on brewing method.

Caffeine-containing products often lack correct and/or adequate information regarding their effects. No Doz, an

OTC stimulant available in the United States, contains only one ingredients—100 mg of caffeine per pill. However, the manufacturer claims that No Doz is non-habit-forming. In fact, this may not be true. Caffeine use leads to dependence— a condition in which the body has adapted to certain daily levels of caffeine and, in fact, has come to depend on them. When caffeine levels abruptly drop, the body reacts, producing withdrawal symptoms characterized by uncomfortable headaches. Therefore, any products containing caffeine—including painkillers and cold remedies—have the potential to be habit-forming.

Ephedrine

Ephedrine, widely used in Chinese folk medicine, was introduced to the West in 1924. It is a *sympathomimetic* drug, which means that it mimics sympathetic nerve stimulation. The sympathetic nervous system elicits responses of alert-

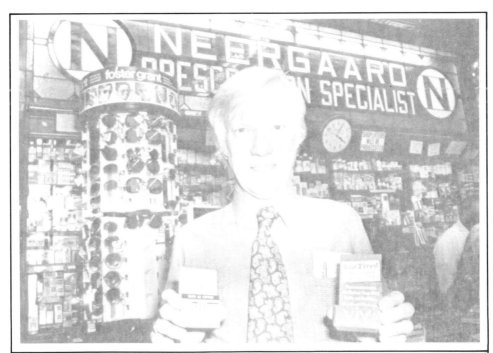

The owner of an all-night pharmacy displays packages of caffeine-containing No Doz and Viv, which reportedly sell well between midnight and 5 A.M. High doses of caffeine can be extremely toxic.

ness, excitement and alarm, and controls the expenditure of energy necessary during an emergency. Sympathetic activation increases heart rate and raises the blood flow to the muscles. The blood vessels supplying the skin and stomach muscles constrict since these parts of the body are not needed to deal with an emergency. And finally, sympathetic activation stimulates the brain so that a person can think and react more quickly. Compared to caffeine, ephedrine's stimulant properties are much more pronounced.

Ephedrine is still used primarily to alleviate the symptoms of asthma (see Chapter 2). Asthma sufferers who ingest ephedrine three to four times a day commonly experience anxiety, agitation, tremulousness and insomnia. This drug has also been linked to heart disease and cerebral haemorrhage (bleeding). In very high doses ephedrine, like amphetamine, is capable of producing psychoses.

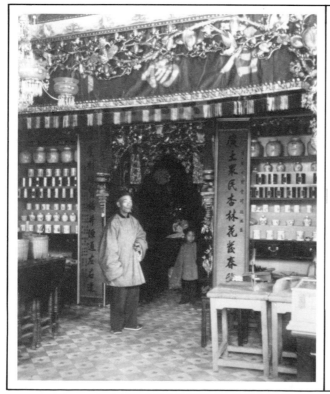

A pharmacy in San Francisco's Chinatown. Like many other drugs used today, ephedrine, a sympathetic-nerve stimulator, was originally discovered centuries ago by the Chinese and widely used in folk medicine.

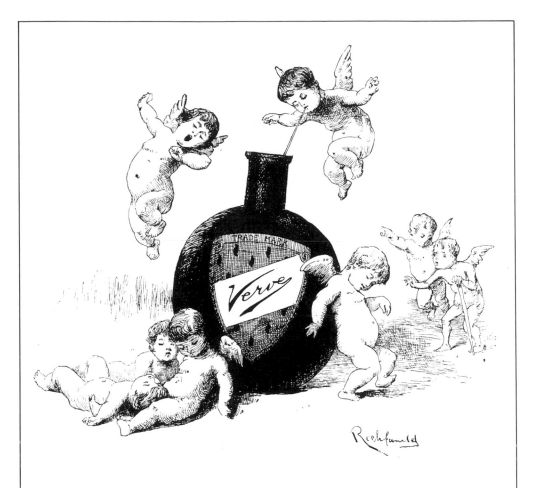

DO YOU SLEEP?

INSOMNIA, the great curse of the American people, is the direct result of Nervous Exhaustion, consequent upon Overwork, Worry, and Mental Strain. The common recourse of the sufferer, is to Opium, Morphine, Chloral, Valerian, Phosphorus, and other drugs whose continued use is fatal.

VERVE contains none of these substances. It is purely vegetable, acts directly upon the exhausted nerve centres, and by its tonic action, produces a healthful, natural sleep, with no after effects. Two or three bottles have cured permanently cases of Insomnia, of months' standing. In Neuralgia, Nervous Irritability, Headache, Mental Depression, Hysteria, Loss of Energy following overwork or continued excitement, and all diseases of the Nervous system it is of inestimable value. Merchants and Business men, Clergymen, Lawyers, Authors, and all persons subject to long-continued mental labor, will find natural sleep easily at hand with this remedy in their possession.

A 19th-century magazine advertisement for "Verve", a "purely vegetable" sleeping medicine safer than narcotics. The manufacturer warns that the continued use of drugs like opium and morphine—which were at the time OTC medications—could be fatal.

CHAPTER 5

RELIEF FROM ANXIETY AND INSOMNIA

About one-third of one's life is spent sleeping. A good night's sleep is crucial to good health, emotional stability, and intellectual clarity. Yet, approximately 30% of all people complain about having difficulty falling asleep and/or staying asleep for a normal duration of time. This condition can have a multitude of causes, such as anxiety, stress, depression, excitation, indigestion or illness. Anxiety can also interfere with one's normal daily activity. Sleeping pills and antianxiety agents may help to alleviate the symptoms of anxiety or insomnia, but if the symptoms continue, the underlying psychological and/or physiological cause(s) should be treated by a professional.

Initially, sleeping pills and antianxiety drugs were relatively easy to obtain with a doctor's prescription. However, in the past ten to fifteen years, scientists and physicians have become more aware of the health hazards and high abuse potential of these drugs. In many countries, prescribing regulations have become tighter and doctors have changed their prescribing habits. As a result it has become more difficult to procure them.

Benzodiazepines (e.g. Valium, Librium) and barbiturates (e.g. Nembutal) are potent relievers of anxiety and insomnia. Prescriptions for Valium and especially barbiturates are more difficult to secure today than they were fifteen or even ten years ago. In most countries, the number of prescriptions for barbiturates decreased substantially during the early 1970s a decline that was partly precipitated by the realization that barbiturates were frequently abused and highly addictive. In fact, barbiturates are often employed by people attempting suicide.

Although the "minor" tranquillizers benzodiazepines and meprobamate (known as Miltown) are safer than the barbiturates, they can cause psychological and physical dependence. In overdose, both the barbiturates and the minor tranquillizers, when taken alone or in conjunction with alcohol, depress brain activity, which can lead to death. As with the barbiturates, after the potential dangers of the minor tranquillizers were more clearly delineated, the number of prescriptions for them has dropped substantially in many countries since the mid-1970s. The increasing reluctance of physicians to prescribe these drugs is well founded.

The Misuse of OTC Sleeping Aids

Today there is an enormous demand for sedation and for

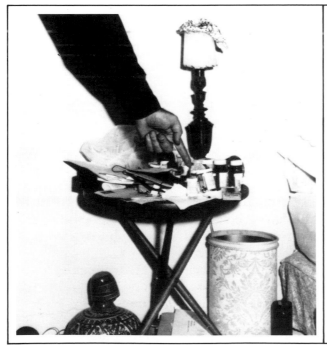

A collection of empty pill bottles on Marilyn Monroe's bedside table. The popular star, who had become increasingly dependent on barbiturates, died from an overdose in August 1962. Most authorities called her death a suicide.

relief from anxiety and insomnia. Pharmaceutical companies have been quick to promote OTC products that supposedly fill this demand, as the American experience demonstrates. After finding that no OTC daytime anxiety reliever or sedative was safe or effective when used for this purpose, the Food and Drugs Administration published regulations in 1979 prohibiting the sale of these products.

In reaction, manufacturers quickly repackaged products, such as Compoz and Quiet World, so they could be sold as sleeping aids.

Although the FDA ruled that no OTC drug can be advertised as anxiety reducing, sleeping aids are used, or, more appropriately, are abused for this purpose. For most products marketed as sleeping aids it is difficult to distinguish between those that are really anxiety relievers and those that are actual sleeping aids. This is due partly to the fact that many consumers believe that a sleeping aid will also relieve daytime anxiety. They understand that too much anxiety, restlessness, or agitation can cause the inability to fall asleep; and since these drugs reduce the night-time anxiety, they

Health experts point out that Americans are among the healthiest people in the world. Pharmaceutical companies, however, spend hundreds of millions of dollars a year to convince consumers that they may have hitherto unsuspected problems, all of which can be easily relieved by the use of "non-habit-forming" drugs.

conclude that they also may be used as daytime anxiety relievers. The manufacturer of Tranquil-Span , for example, states outright that this drug "helps calm and relax you", and only indirectly ties this statement to also helping you fall asleep. The name Tranquil-Span itself implies an anxiety-free period of time, and not necessarily sleep. Thus it should not be surprising that these drugs are misused as anxiety relievers.

Antihistamines

Antihistamines, a major ingredient in cold remedies, are also found in sleeping aids. Pyrilamine maleate, diphenhydramine hydrochloride (HCI) and, to a lesser extent, doxylamine succinate are the most common antihistamines used to produce drowsiness. Two of these antihistamines, diphenhydramine HCI and doxylamine succinate, were changed from prescription to nonprescription drugs within the past few years. Some manufacturers also include analgesics such as aspirin or paracetamol in their sleeping-aid products just in case pain, such as a headache or backache, is a factor causing insomnia.

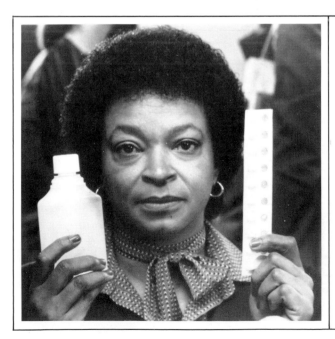

Two types of child-resistant drug packaging. These are recommended for products containing antihistamines, which can be dangerous if misused.

Although brand names often remain constant over a period of years, the ingredients in any particular brand may change frequently. This practice makes it difficult to evaluate and compare OTC products in an intelligent way. Clearly, manufacturers are not very interrested in educating the consumer to do this.

Anticholinergics

Until a few years ago, the anticholinergics scopolamine and atropine were also sold alone or in combination with antihistamines for relief from anxiety and insomnia. They are effective for this purpose because, in addition to drying up runny noses (see Chapter 2), the anticholinergic drugs cause

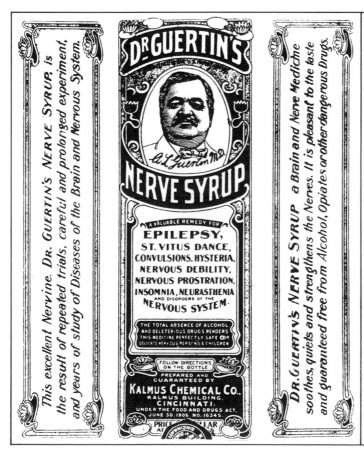

A typical patent medicine, "Dr. Guertin's Nerve Syrup" promised relief for a wide variety of complaints. Such products enjoyed enormous popularity in the 19th and early 20th centuries. One advertisement contained a sworn testimonial from a customer who said, "I am satisfied that my life has been preserved and my health entirely restored."

drowsiness and sedation. However, they also cause side effects such as a dry mouth, nose and throat, blurred vision, ringing ears, upset stomach, decreased appetite and thickened bronchial secretions. Elderly people are likely to experience dizziness and confusion, and men may have trouble in initiating urination, especially if they have an enlarged prostate gland. At higher doses, nervousness, tremors, muscle spasms, and even convulsions may occur. And hallucinations, heart palpitations, headaches and, paradoxically, insomnia are also not uncommon. Because of the prominence of these undesirable effects, the OTC sale of anticholinergics is prohibited in many countries.

Combination Products

In 1979 it was common to encounter methapyrilene (an antihistamine) and scopolamine (an anticholinergic) in the same sleep aid. Although these drugs are no longer

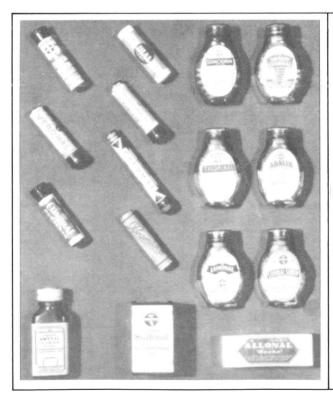

"Synthetic sleep" products available in the 1930s were based on formulas devloped in Germany and seized by U.S. authorities after World War I. The principal ingredient in all the preparations was Veronal, the first barbiturate, which had been introduced in 1903.

manufactured, people who purchased them previously may still have them in their medicine cabinets.

Unfortuately, once people discovered that these drugs could get you high, they were abused. The synergism (when two drugs together produce effects greater than either one alone) of anticholinergic and antihistaminergic effects, magnified by the ingestion of very high doses, created effects which, though rarely fatal, were not uncommonly associated with drug-induced psychosis. This condition was characterized by hallucinations, confusion, disorientation, delirium and agitation, or hyperactivity. Drastically increased heart rate (as high as 140 beats per minute), hypertension and varying degrees of coma are also common effects associated with the abuse of these substances. A 1977 report in a scientific journal described five deaths that were directly attributable to these products.

Advertising

The sleeping aids that are still being sold have the potential to be dangerous. As mentioned above, they all contain anti-histamines, some of which have already been proved to be

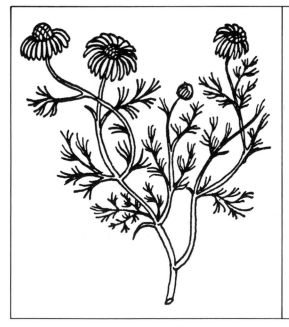

One does not need to rely on potentially dangerous drugs to treat insomnia. Camomile tea, made from the flowers of the herb Anthemis nobilis *is a natural sedative and anxiety reliever. Hot milk, drunk just before going to bed, increases sleep time and decreases night-time restlessness. And exercise done early in the day dramatically improves sleep.*

ineffective and/or unsafe. While these drugs were designed to treat alleregic reactions, their use as a sleeping aid is based solely on their side effect of producing drowsiness in some people.

People continue to use these drugs simply because drug companies continue their advertising campaigns. In 1977 Bristol-Myers, one of the largest pharmaceutical companies in the world, spent over 114 million dollars on television advertising in America, while General Motors (the world's largest automobile manufacturing company) spent about 91 million dollars. The drug companies realize that by repeatedly emphasizing a drug's benefits, not only does the

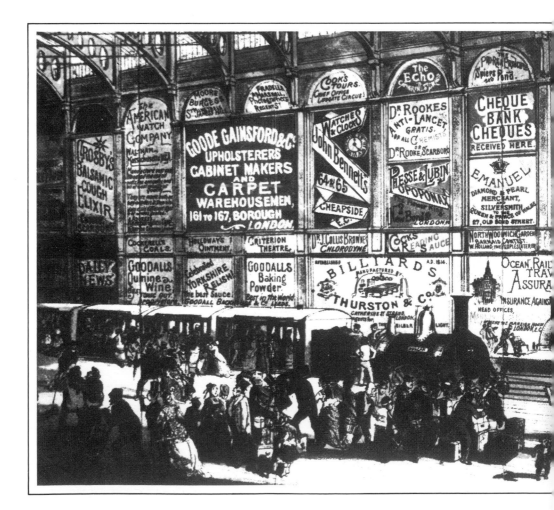

consumer come to believe the advertisment, but this belief greatly increases the chances that the product will, in fact, be effective. This placebo effect (see Chapter 6) greatly increases the success of the advertising campaigns, which causes a steady rise in sales.

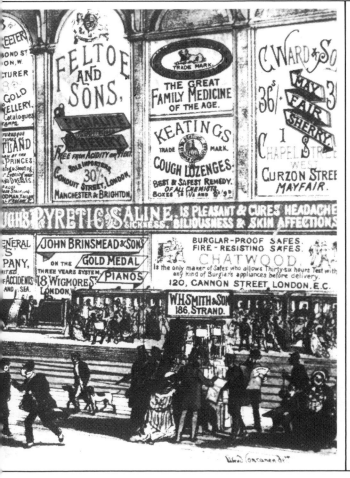

Saturation advertising techniques are not new, as this view of a London railway station in 1874 demonstrates. The posters that dominate the space extol the virtues of everything from carpets and baking powder to a medicine that guarantees to cure "headache, biliousness and skin affections".

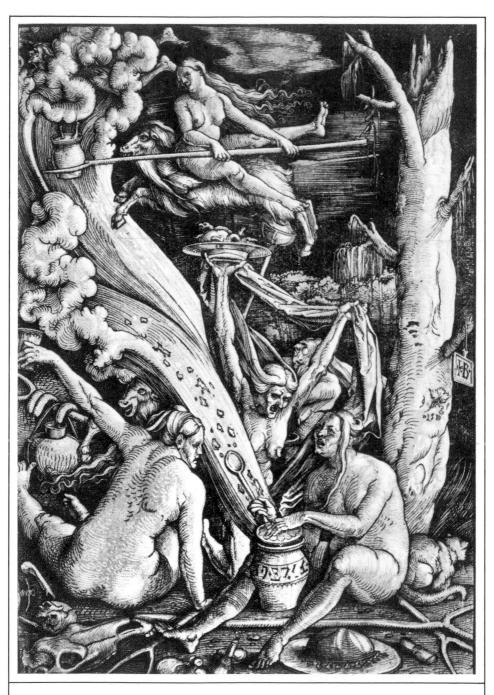

Witches' Sabbath, *a 15th-century woodcut. Medieval belief in the supernatural was so powerful that people sometimes fell ill when they believed they had received the curse of a witch.*

CHAPTER 6

PLACEBO

*S*ince the beginning of recorded history, flyspecks, snake flesh, mummy powder, asses' hooves, crocodile droppings, and frog sperm have produced many a wonderous cure for even the most stubborn of ailments. One can only speculate on what people may have used as medicine before this time. But, as time went on, the physicians' remedies became a trifle more sophisticated. For example, Thomas Jefferson once wrote to a friend that, "One of the most successful physicians I have ever known has assured me that he used more of bread pills, drops of coloured water, and powders of hickory ashes than all other medicines put together."

Most of these concoctions worked because of a phenomenon known as the *placebo effect*. It was first alluded to in published form by Robert Burton in 1628: "An empiric oftentimes, and a silly chirurgeon, doth more strange cures than a rational physician ... because his patient puts his confidence in him." Near the end of the 18th century Benjamin Franklin led a commission to investigate this phenomenon. The commission concluded that the patient's imagination was responsible for the bizarre occurrences, and the unbelievable cures were not a result of mesmerization per se. In fact, contrary to popular belief, no scientific study has furnished conclusive proof that the occurrence of the placebo effect is related to the suggestibility of an individual at all.

One definition of placebo is "a preparation, devoid of pharmacological effect, given for psychological effect, or as a control in evaluating a medicine believed to have pharmacological activity". The word placebo is derived from Latin, meaning "I shall please". And this is exactly what placebos are meant to do.

Because of a patient's trust in his or her doctor, placebos may have significant effects. This is no different from trusting a television commercial, a magazine advertisement, or word of mouth. Once a doctor or a television actor has a person's trust, he or she may be easily convinced of the effectiveness of whatever product is being "sold." The manner in which the medication is given and the setting in which it is administered also contribute to the overall effect. Thus, in effect, watching a television advertisment in which a very compassionate wife gives her husband a cold remedy, and receiving medicine from your own sympathetic doctor are much the same.

Some OTC products depend almost exclusively on the placebo effect since many such drugs are entirely ineffective for treatment of the illness for which they are intended. Yet, products that have been shown to have no pharmacological effect are still on the market, and people continue to buy them. Perhaps they know something that the clinical tests have not shown. It is likely that the actual benefits associated with these drugs are due to the placebo effect.

Doctors knowingly use placebos more than most

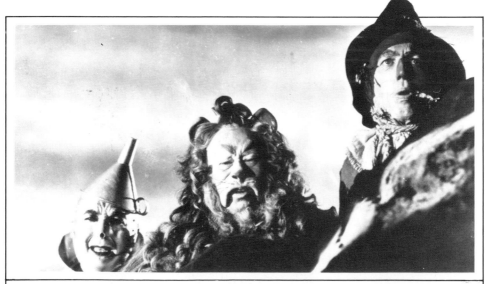

In the film **The Wizard of Oz,** *the Tin Man got a pocket watch that ticked and felt he had a heart; the Cowardly Lion was awarded a medal for courage and became brave; and the Scarecrow was given a diploma and knew he had a brain. All three cases are examples of the placebo effect.*

patients are aware. How does a patient actually know that a drug is working because of its pharmacological action and not its placebo effect? One way to answer this question is to test a drug in a *double-blind* experiment.

Double-Blind Studies

Because the placebo effect can be very strong and is responsible for a significant percentage of a drug's therapeutic efficacy, new pharmacological substances are today routinely tested in double-blind experiments.

A double-blind study compares the efficacy of a drug with that of a placebo. One-half of the patients are given the pharmacologically inert (ineffective) placebo and the other half receive the drug; but neither the doctors, nurses, nor patients know who received what until the study is concluded. This is referred to as double-blind because both groups, the patients and the judges, are "blind" as to who receives a drug and who receives a placebo.

Because it has been shown that the doctor's faith in a drug's curative power has a marked effect on the patient's

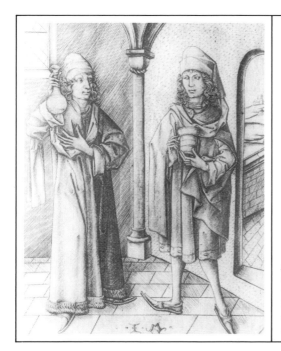

Cosmas (left) was a 3rd-century physician, and his brother Damian was an apothecary. Christian missionaries and martyrs, they became the patron saints, respectively, of doctors and druggists.

perception of the drug's effectiveness, it is important to ensure that this confidence in the new drug does not influence the results of the study. Keeping the doctor in the dark ensures that he or she will treat both the drug and the placebo in the same fashion. And the patient's desire for a favourable outcome from the treatment thereby increases the possibility that *both* placebo and drug are effective. Thus, any positive or negative effects can be attributed only to the action of the drug.

Impure Placebos

Placebos are described as being pure (a sugar pill or a saline injection, both of which have no pharmacological action) and impure (vitamin B_{12} or penicillin, when used to treat an illness for which they have no effect). Because of vitamin B_{12}'s limited pharmacological activity and low cost it is probably the most popular placebo prescribed by doctors. In the years 1980 and 1981, of 1.2 billion visits to the doctor in the United States, 8 million resulted in a B_{12} prescription for patients who had no symptoms that B_{12} could have affected at all.

Most OTC preparations fall in the impure placebo category. Studies have repeatedly found that impure placebos are generally more successful than pure, or totally inert, substances in producing the suggested subjective effect in the patient. For example, patients who are suffering from anxiety may be given a drug that does affect their physiology (e.g., causes light-headedness, dry mouth, and/or dilated pupils) or one that has no effect at all. If they are told in both cases that they will feel relaxed, it is likely that they will feel more relaxed after taking the drug that has some kind of physiological action. It is possible that any noticeable effects are interpreted by the patient as being related to the desired subjective experience, in this case relaxation. Or perhaps any change in their internal state is perceived as being beneficial.

As long as a drug has some effect its other placebo-type effects will actually amplify the main effect. OTC drugs depend on this phenomenon to a large extent. Antihistamines, apart from blocking inflammation due to histamine release, have a dozen or so other effects. What may be called a side effect when the drug is used for one purpose may be a main effect when the drug is used for another purpose. Advertisements select and focus on the effect they want to be noticed. This is why when advertisers repeatedly state that their product will aid sleep, there is a good chance that it will.

This concept plays a highly important role in the use and abuse of legal, illegal, nonprescription and prescription drugs. If a teenager's best friend tells him that if he takes two "black beauties" he will get high and feel just great all night long, as long as the drug produces some physiological signs of euphoria his friend's assertions could boost a mild experience to a great high.

Pure Placebos

Pure placebos are also capable of affecting physiology. They may cause changes in blood pressure, heart rate, blood cell counts, creatinine and lipoprotein levels, respiratory rate, pupil size, body temperature, gastrointestinal secretions and bowel movements. It is surprising what a sugar pill can do if given by the right person and under the proper conditions.

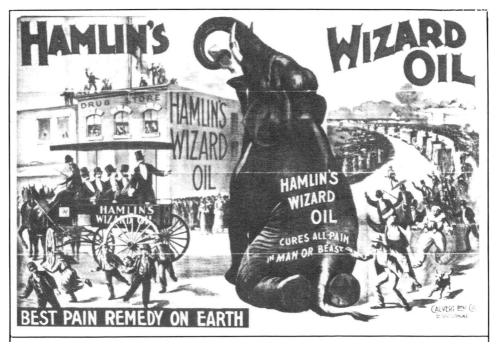

"Wizard Oil" was one of the 19th century's most popular OTC placebos.

The pain-relieving effects of placebos have been the most widely studied and are the most well established. Since the brain does not differentiate between "imagined" pain (that caused by mental events) and "real" pain (that caused by the activation of pain receptors in the body), placebo treatments are just as effective in relieving both types. *Endorphins,* chemicals found in the brain, are now well recognized as the body's own painkillers. They act in the same way as opiates such as morphine or codeine. When one is given a placebo and told it is a very effective pain-killer, endorphins are released and have a significant pain-relieving effect.

Thus, placebos do much more than just make people think they are better. Whenever a person unknowingly ingests an inert placebo when he or she is expecting an effect, thirty to forty per cent of the time that effect is apt to occur. And sometimes the expected or desired effect is accompanied by the same side effects associated with the ingestion of the pharmacologically active drug. There is no such thing as a harmless drug or a perfectly harmless placebo.

Size, Shape and Colour

Studies designed to clarify the relationship between form (capsule or tablet), size, shape and colour of pills have provided some interesting results. In most cases the larger the tablet or capsule, the greater the placebo effect. This is supported by the fact that capsules which are larger than, though pharmacologically equal to, tablets are usually perceived as being stronger than tablets.

Most interesting are recent findings correlating the colour of the pill and the anticipated effect. Yellow, orange and, to some small extent, bright red and black are most often associated with stimulants or antidepressants. On the other hand, white is mostly associated with analgesics and narcotics. This type of information is frequently used by drug manufacturers, both to promote sales and to increase the effectiveness of drugs.

Placebos: Pros and Cons

Many physicians feel that the use of placebos is deceitful and therefore unethical. They argue that they "can heal just as well without deception". They also state that the use of placebos perpetuates quackery, since quacks depend heavily on placebos.

It can be argued that there is nothing wrong with a white lie that persuades the patient to purchase a much less expensive placebo prescription if it has the same effects as a more expensive drug. One cannot ignore the fact that even the strongest drugs have placebo effects that are diminished or enhanced by various stimuli only indirectly related to the drug itself. Many people are very drug-oriented and are more likely to opt for a quick medical cure than for a healthier, preventive life style. But clearly, if the supply of placebos and many OTC drugs were to be completely denied to the public, people would be forced to seek alternatives within a new mode of living.

When a doctor prescribes a placebo, he or she hopefully has the patient's best interest in mind. In the case of an advertisement, however, the motivation is more likely to be financial. And yet, the advertisements are not totally misleading—even placebos are beneficial thirty to forty per cent of the time. This distinction between deception of and deceit against the public is a very fine one, but as long as people continue to rely heavily on the continued use of these drugs to feel better and to cope with everyday life, OTC products will undoubtedly remain on the market.

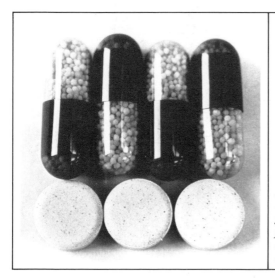

Extended-release capsules, with their hundreds of individual grains of medication, are usually perceived as being more potent than tablets, even when they are of equal strength.

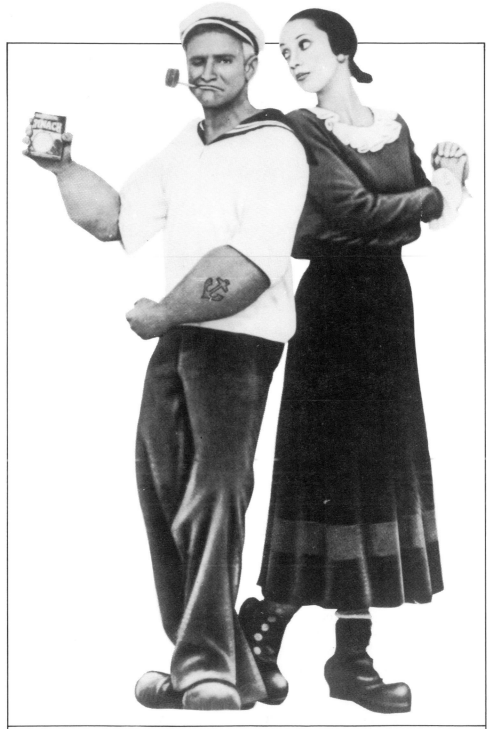

In the movie Popeye, *the comic-strip spinach-eating sailor had the right idea. When cooked briefly, spinach is an excellent source of vitamins A, E, K, C, B_1 (thiamine), B_2 (riboflavin) and niacin.*

CHAPTER 7

NUTRITIONAL SUPPLEMENTS

Because vitamins are not considered drugs, they can be marketed in the United States without Food and Drug Administration control. This alone is probably part of the reason why vitamins and related products outsell every other category of OTC products. In 1981 sales of nutritional products (just less than 2 billion dollars) were more than twice as great as those of the next two highest sellers—analgesics and cold remedies. In 1984 the figures for vitamin sales were far in excess of 2 billion dollars. Americans have been growing increasingly aware of the importance of proper nutrition, partly because of wide coverage by the media, and partly because of the growing realization by the medical profession that a good diet is essential to good health. The old adage "you are what you eat" is probably more true than people ever realized.

With the pace of life ever increasing, many people have become dependent on 10-minute meals so as not to waste too much time. To make sure that our bodies remain capable of functioning more or less normally, we take Alka Seltzer to treat indigestion and mega-vitamins to provide the other ingredients our meal may have lacked. Mega-vitamins are pills that contain one or more vitamins in amounts ten or more times the Recommended Daily Allowance (Table 4).

Popular literature extols the virtues of taking vitamin supplements in mega-doses. The supposed benefits include the prevention of cancer, increased sexual prowess, pre-

Table 4

Recommended Daily Allowances		
NUTRIENT	MALES	FEMALES
Vitamin C (mg)	60	60
Thiamine (mg)	1.4	1.0
Riboflavin (mg)	1.6	1.2
Niacin (mg)	18	13
Vitamin B_6 (mg)	2.2	2.0
Folacin (μg)	400	400
Vitamin B_{12} (μg)	3.0	3.0
Vitamin A (μg)	1000	800
Vitamin D (μg)	5	5
Vitamin E (mg)	10	8

SOURCE: U.S. Food and Nutrition Board, National Academy of Sciences, National Research Council Committee on Dietary Allowances, 1980. Recommended for healthy adults ages 23-50. May vary for other age groups, during pregnancy and lactation. Official recommendations for vitamin K, biotin, or pantothenic acid have not been established.

vention or cure of the common cold, retardation of the aging process, increased capability to handle stress, and prevention and cure of mental illness.

Diets centred around multiple vitamins and minerals in mega-doses have been the focus of investigations of practically every type of mental illness. This type of therapy is referred to as *orthomolecular psychiatry*. Most commonly included in such a regimen are niacin, vitamin C, pyridoxine, vitamin E and vitamin B_{12}. Claims include the cure and even prevention of schizophrenia, neurosis, depression, alcoholism, hyperactivity and autism. However, these claims do not stand up in double-blind studies.

The term "vitamin" carries with it the connotation of well-being and health. Although vitamins are essential and generally beneficial to our health, many people do not really appreciate their true function. Of the thousands of substances that the human body needs in order to function properly, there are 47 that the human body cannot synthesize from other compounds and thus have to be supplied by the food we eat. Of these 47, thirteen are vitamins.

The function of vitamins was first realized around the turn of the century. Ever since then vitamins, at least in the public's eye, have been acquiring ever-increasing magical powers. Practically all claims of cures or prophylaxis (prevention) are illogically based on the reversal of symptoms accompanying special vitamin deficiencies. For example, vitamin E has been lauded as a veritable guarantor of male virility and sexual prowess. This is based on the fact that vitamin E deficiency causes sterility in male laboratory rats. If these rats are given sufficient amounts of vitamin E within a certain period of time, then the sterility is reversed. To date there is no significant evidence that would corroborate assertions that high vitamin E intake will increase sexual function to above normal levels.

This type of faulty reasoning forms the basis of many arguments put forward by proponents of mega-vitamin therapy. The examples that follow should further clarify this point. Despite the inaccuracy of vitamin-related information, one should keep in mind that compared to all the other substances discussed in this book, vitamins actually have the least potential to do any harm. Nonetheless, this is not to say that they can do no harm.

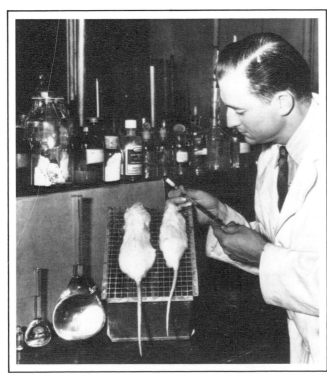

Laboratory rats wait for their daily dose of B$_{12}$. One gram of B$_{12}$ supplies the daily requirements of twenty million rats, and one-millionth of a gram per day will treat pernicious anaemia in humans.

In the 1980s the quantities of vitamins being ingested by the general population are more than alarming. The fact that the media are successfully convincing us that eating "alphabet soup" in pill form is beneficial has created a new kind of drug-abuse problem.

Vitamins are most practically divided into water-soluble or fat-soluble. Since the body quickly excretes and does not store water-soluble vitamins, they are virtually harmless. However, because fat-soluble vitamins are stored in fat cells (lipid tissue), and therefore remain in the body for much longer, they have much greater potential for toxicity.

Water-Soluble Vitamins

Vitamin C, or ascorbic acid, is the most widely renowned water-soluble vitamin. It is also the vitamin most frequently used in mega-doses. Because it is so popular, more is known about its use than that of any of the other vitamins. Though it has a reputation as a prophylactic and as a cure for the common cold, tests nearly conclusively show that it will not prevent the occurrence of a cold; however, it might decrease the severity and duration of the infection. To achieve this effect, however, the daily mega-doses of 500 mg–2,000 mg frequently taken by many individuals are not required. In fact, supplements of even less than 100 mg per day are

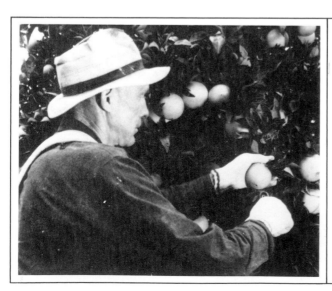

An orange picker inspects his crop. Though oranges are the best-known sources of vitamin C, it is also available in such fruits as papayas, stawberries, mangoes and cantaloupes, and in such vegetables as tomatoes, broccoli and Brussels sprouts.

sufficient. This amount is found in a glass of orange juice.

Apart from its supposed effect on the common cold, vitamin C has also been asserted to be effective treatment for many viral, bacterial and fungal infections. There is, however, no reliable evidence for this.

Daily intake of large doses of vitamin C has also been recommended for the prevention of post-transfusion hepatitis (inflammation of the liver), venous thrombosis (clotting of the blood in a vein), some of the complications associated with diabetes mellitus, lung damage from air pollution (including smoking), and sudden infant death. It is also purported to enhance the healing of wounds and to increase altertness, overall mental capability and the ability to cope with stress. Of these claims very few are substantiated.

There is reason to believe that vitamin C may be beneficial in guarding against venous thrombosis, but evidence is not yet conclusive. The claim that vitamin C is beneficial in the healing of wounds is based on its importance in the formation of *collagen,* a fibrous protein found in bone, cartilage and connective tissue which is involved in the process of wound healing. Furthermore there is evidence that high vitamin C intake is of therapeutic value in the treatment of corneal burns. However, scientific proof is lacking to support similar wound-healing properties in any other bodily tissues.

Even with massive doses, vitamin C rarely causes adverse reactions. There are exceptions, however. Vitamin C used in excess of 1000 mg per day has been associated with diarrhoea, gastrointestinal irritation and abdominal cramps. Part of this is due to the fact that vitamin C is an acid, hence its name, ascorbic acid. The possibility of forming gallstones (nephrolithiasis) is apparently increased with high doses, especially in individuals already predisposed to this illness.

Whenever any substance is given to an organism in abnormally high amounts, the metabolic processes that utilize that substance are altered—generally accelerated to deal with the increased amounts. If the supply of the substance suddenly returns to the normal level, the metabolic processes for that substance are still set for the previous high level, and the substance is therefore metabolized and excreted at the previous high rate. This results in a net deficiency of that substance.

If mega-doses of vitamin C are suddenly halted, the symptoms associated with vitamin C deficiency can occur. The only serious vitamin C withdrawal symptom is scurvy. Scurvy is characterized by weakness, spongy gums, anaemia, and bleeding of the mucous membranes. Because pregnant women are made very aware of the fact that the presence or absence of practically anything in their bodies is going to affect their baby, many try to guarantee their baby's health by taking mega-vitamins. Doing this with vitamin C will cause "rebound scurvy" in the newborn, if, after the child is born the mega-doses of vitamin C are no longer made available.

B vitamins are popular because of their alleged role in preventing and alleviating stress-related problems. The B-complex vitamins include thiamine (B_1), riboflavin (B_2), niacin, pyridoxine (B_6), folic acid, B_{12}, pantothenic acid and biotin. A number of other substances are also frequently commercialized under the B-complex rubric, though they really do not belong there. These include choline, inositol, para-aminobenzoic acid (PABA), orotic acid (B_{13}), pargamic

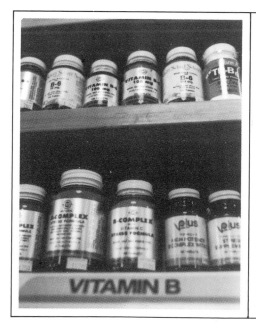

Health-food store shelves are crowded with pills and capsules containing vitamin B complex, which is actually thirteen separate vitamins. A well-balanced diet provides most people with adequate B vitamins, but pregnant women, children and individuals who ingest excessive amounts of carbohydrates may need extra vitamin B.

acid (B_{15}), and laetrile (B_{17}). Some are included because they are growth factors (e.g., choline and inositol); others, such as orotic acid and laetrile, have no basis for inclusion as either growth factors or vitamins. Orotic acid is a co-enzyme in the biosynthetic pathway of nucleotides (which are important substances in the formation of DNA and RNA), whereas laetrile includes a group of related organic substances obtained from plants. There is as yet no conclusive evidence that laetrile plays any significant role in animal metabolism or in the cure for cancer (as popularly believed).

Thiamine is supposedly capable of relieving depression, anxiety and mental illness, as well as preventing senility. It has no known adverse effects when taken orally.

Riboflavin is proclaimed to ensure healthier skin, nails and hair and to improve vision. It also has no known negative effects.

Niacin, which comes in the form of nicotinic acid or nicotinamide, is associated with significant pharmacological effects and has therefore been studied quite extensively. Although it is effective as a fat-lowering agent in people suffering from hyperlipemia (an excess of fat or lipids in the blood), it has no weight-reducing effects on people not

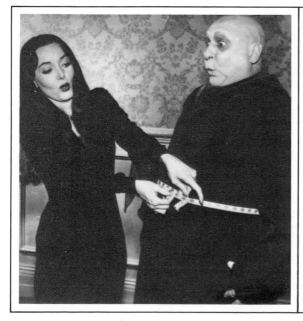

Morticia in **The Addams Family** *evaluating Uncle Fester's weight loss. For those people who suffer from hyperlipemia (an excess of fat in the blood), niacin has proved to be effective as a fat-lowering agent.*

suffering from this disease. There is also no proof that it is beneficial in reducing cholesterol levels. The most common side effects are flushing of the face, neck and chest and cardiac arrhythmias (abnormal heart beats). However, even at relatively low doses (100 mg–300 mg) both nicotinamide and nicotinic acid use can lead to headaches, cramps, nausea, vomiting, diarrhoea, hypotension, and hypoglycaemia. At higher doses, the major concern is hepatotoxicity.

Vitamin B$_6$ (pyridoxine, pyridoxal, and pyridoxamine) is of concern because contraceptive-induced abnormalities are reversible with vitamin B$_6$ supplementation. In addition, a number of cases have been reported in which increased vitamin B$_6$ intake was effective in alleviating premenstrual tension. However, vitamin B$_6$ is known to cause dependency at doses as low as 200 mg per day.

Folic acid is relatively less popular. It has been used in the treatment of women with a high risk for neural-tube defects in their children. But again, proof of its positive effects is merely circumstantial. Anecdotal evidence suggests that it may decrease the beneficial effects of phenytoin, a chemical used in the treatment of epileptics. The major concern with folic acid is that it masks vitamin B$_{12}$ deficiency.

The possible role in folic acid in mental disorders has

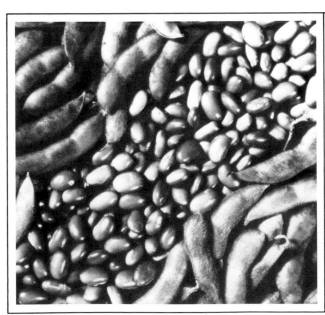

Soybeans, shown here both shelled and unshelled, are rich in protein and folic acid, a vitamin also abundant in other legumes, such as kidney beans, lima beans, white beans and peas. Cultivated in China since before 3500 B.C., the soybean is a versatile and extremely nutritious vegetable and is thirty-five per cent protein.

received considerable attention. In several studies institutionalized mental health patients exhibited abnormally low folic acid levels in twenty to fifty per cent of cases. However, subsequent studies prompted by this finding did not show that patients experienced any consistent improvement following folic acid supplementation.

Vitamin B₁₂. An adult stores about 5 mg of vitamin B_{12} (mainly in the liver) and only about one microgram daily is required to maintain this level. Since many people ingest as much as 85 mg daily, dietary deficiency of vitamin B_{12} is extremely rare. It can only occur after a prolonged, strict vegetarian diet that excludes all meat, eggs and dairy products.

One of the few instances in which vitamin B_{12} supplementation is of benefit is in patients suffering from *pernicious anaemia,* a disorder that prevents the absorption of B_{12} into the blood stream. When it is given intravenously to replenish B_{12} stores, it characteristically results in short-term acne, usually not lasting longer than one week.

Pantothenic acid has no known pharmacologic effects. One study, using human volunteers, reported that it is helpful in coping with the stress of being immersed in cold water. Even at high doses no interactions with other medications or toxicity have been noted.

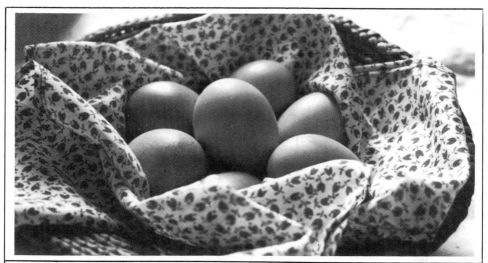

Vegetarians have to worry about vitamin B_{12} deficiency, for this vitamin is most abundant in animal products, such as eggs. Tempeh, an Indonesian soy product, is also a good source of vitamin B_{12}.

Fat-Soluble Vitamins

Vitamins A, D, E and K are fat-soluble vitamins. Since they are stored in the fat cells of the body, rather than being rapidly metabolized and excreted, they have a much greater propensity for causing adverse effects than do water-soluble vitamins. Each of them individually may reach different levels at various times (depending on daily intake and rate of metabolism for each of these vitamins in an individual), and thus they can have something analogous to a "seesaw" effect on one another. If low levels of fat-soluble vitamins are generally present, and only one of them is taken in supranormal amounts, its toxicity will be very noticeable and possibly exaggerated. Conversely, if high or adequate levels of a fat-soluble vitamin are present and a person ingests high levels of another one of these vitamins, no adverse symptoms are noted. For example, high vitamin E concentrations protect against both vitamin A and vitamin D toxicity, and high concentrations of vitamin D protect against symptoms of vitamin A deficiency, and vice versa.

Vitamin A is very popular due to a handful of encouraging, albeit misrepresented, reports. Frequently included in popular literature are claims of vitamin A's prevention of cancer, aid in increasing resistance to a wide variety of ailments and diseases (including acne), and promotion of healthy bones, skin, hair, teeth and gums. Most of these claims are, however, based on very meagre, if any, scientific evidence.

Vitamin A is primarily stored in the liver. Therefore, the major concern with both short- and long-term, high-level intake of vitamin A is its hepatotoxicity. In fact, prolonged mega-doses of vitamin A have been known to result in tender bones, hair loss, bleeding, nausea, vomiting and anorexia. Furthermore, although some current magazine articles claim otherwise, a mega-dose vitamin A intake is definitely not advisable for pregnant mothers. An above-normal incidence of deformations in almost all foetal organ systems has been found to be highly correlated with this type of high vitamin A diet.

Fortunately, in most cases, if normal levels of vitamin A intake are resumed before permanent damage is done,

Table 5

Fat-Soluble Vitamins and Their Sources	
FAT-SOLUBLE VITAMINS	NATURAL SOURCES
Vitamin A Essential for bone formation, healthy skin & mucous membranes.	*Retinol*, found in meat products, and *carotene*, which is found in yellow/orange fruits & vegetables, & leafy green vegetables, including carrots; sweet potatoes; cantaloupe; tomatoes; papaya; red peppers; kale; broccoli.
Vitamin D Essential for bone growth, metabolism of calcium & phosphorus.	Sunshine, eggs, milk & other dairy products.
Vitamin E May counteract respiratory problems caused by air pollution.	Vegetable oils, especially wheat germ, walnut, sunflower & safflower oil; sunflower seeds, almonds, hazelnuts & walnuts; spinach, sweet potatoes, beet & turnip greens.
Vitamin K Necessary for normal clotting of blood.	Leafy green vegetables, egg yolk, soybean oil.

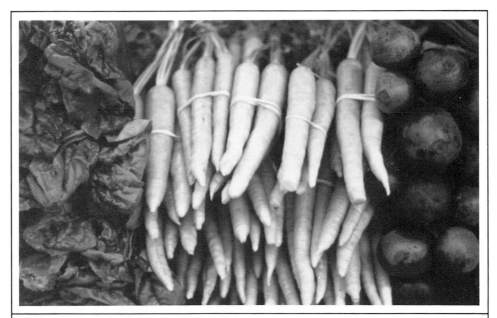

All vitamins occur naturally in foods and are essential for bodily functions. A recent report claimed that "foods rich in carotene, or vitamin A, may lower the risk of cancer".

hepatotoxic reactions associated with high vitamin A levels are reversible.

Vitamin D is probably the least abused vitamin. Because it is known to be extremely toxic, even the lay literature does not promote its use. Its potential for toxicity is almost exclusively rooted in its very prominent role as a regulator of calcium metabolism. It is intimately involved in transporting calcium across the intestinal wall. Abnormally high vitamin D levels cause hypercalcemia—abnormally elevated levels of calcium. This is often characterized by weakness, increased urination, thirst, nausea, anorexia, sleepiness and/or stupor.

In one case a young boy had been ingesting as much as 250,000 IU (international units) of vitamin A and 4,000 IU of vitamin D per day. Finally he suffered from excessive amounts of calcium in the blood, increased intracranial pressure, headaches, rash, fever, swelling of face and limbs due to fluid retention, bone pain and tenderness, and other

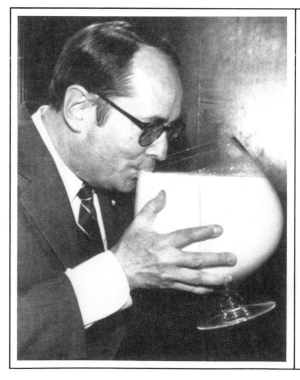

Milk is a superior source of complete protein, as well as of calcium, riboflavin, and vitamin D, which is usually added after the milk has been pasteurized.

symptoms. Fortunately, he recovered after hospitalization.

Children are much more prone to the toxic effects of both vitamin A and D, while adults are relatively resistant. Although daily doses of 10,000 IU per day have resulted in complications after only a few months, usually doses of 50,000 IU–500,000 IU daily over a period of years are required to produce adverse effects in adults.

Vitamin E is probably the next most popular vitamin after vitamin C. It as been marketed and widely sold as a restorer or enhancer of male virility. It is also renowned as a prophylactic and cure for a variety of skin problems. In this area it is credited with speeding up the healing process of nearly any kind of superficial wound, as well as being able to create a healthy skin tone. There is reliable scientific data that conclusively supports these claims. Vitamin E has also been widely acclaimed as a cure for fibrocystic breast disease, an abnormal increase of fibrous connective tissue in the breast. Again, no conclusive data are available.

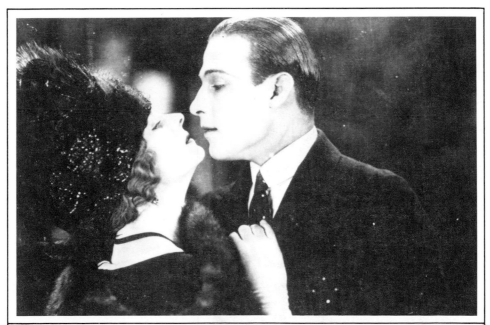

Rudolph Valentino (1895-1926) demonstrates the passionate look that made him the 1920s' best-known male sex symbol. The silent-film star was said to use aphrodisiacs in an effort to boost his sexual powers.

Ever since 1946, when vitamin E gained a reputation as being useful in treating angina pectoris (recurrent pain in the chest and left arm caused by a sudden decrease of the blood supply to the heart), rumours of its curative powers have increased. Now they include prevention and treatment of many heart-related problems, including myocardial infarctions, rheumatic heart disease, congenital heart disease and congestive heart failure. However, mega-doses of vitamin E have not yet been proved to have therapeutic value in any type of cardiovascular disorder.

In the 1980s vitamin E is still acclaimed as a virtual guarantee for a normal pregnancy. This claim, however, is based on individual cases from the 1940s and 1950s, when women known to spontaneously abort were given mega-vitamin E treatment. Even in these cases the improvement was only marginal and not statistically significant.

Vitamin E has been shown to relieve pain and limping due to peripheral vascular occlusion (i.e., the closing of superficial blood vessels, usually those supplying the leg muscles). And its possible prophylactic effects on athero-

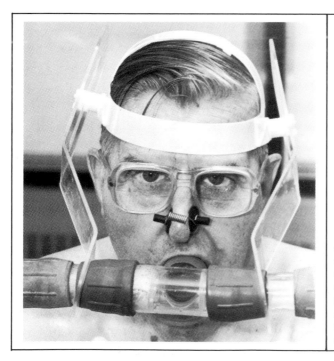

Wearing a nose clamp and a mouthpiece that analyzes his exhaled breath as he exercises, a volunteer takes part in a study aimed at learning how diet and vitamin intake affect the aging process.

sclerosis (a degenerative disease of the arteries) have been noted. Apparently vitamin E redistributes cholesterol stores in such a way that high concentrations of cholesterol in a limited area become unlikely, and therefore the chances of developing atherosclerosis are minimized.

There are also claims of vitamin E preventing thrombophlebitis (inflammation of a vein associated with, or due to, a thrombus, or a blood clot). In fact, most of the above-mentioned claims are conjectural, and based mostly on scattered reports of individual cases and on unreplicated studies. The possibility does exist that in the future some of these effects will be supported by substantial evidence.

Modern-day living exposes us to higher than normal amounts of ozone, nitrogen oxide and a wide variety of other air pollutants. Vitamin E has, in fact, shown some efficacy in ameliorating respiratory problems associated with this situation.

In a 1974 study, 82% of sufferers of nocturnal leg cramps (50% of which had experienced the symptom for more than five years) benefited from doses of vitamin E.

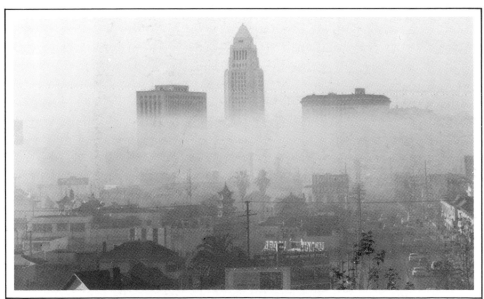

A thermal inversion, or layer of warm air that traps polluted air beneath it, hovers over Los Angeles. Some medical researchers believe that vitamin E can ease respiratory problems caused by such conditions.

Although vitamin E, being a fat-soluble vitamin, remains in the body for prolonged periods of time, very large daily amounts have rarely been the cause of health problems. Nevertheless, there have been reports of skin eruptions, muscle weakness and stomachache associated with daily mega-doses (100 IU–1,000 IU) of vitamin E.

Vitamin K, an essential agent involved in blood coagulation, is easily obtained in effective amounts from a more or less normal diet. No serious side effects attributable to mega-doses of vitamin K have as yet been reported.

Because vitamins and other essential nutrients, due to their relatively benign pharmacologic and toxic effects, have traditionally been viewed as undeserving of serious consideration, we in fact know relatively little about them. Therefore, all claims, even those backed by some scientific evidence, should be taken lightly.

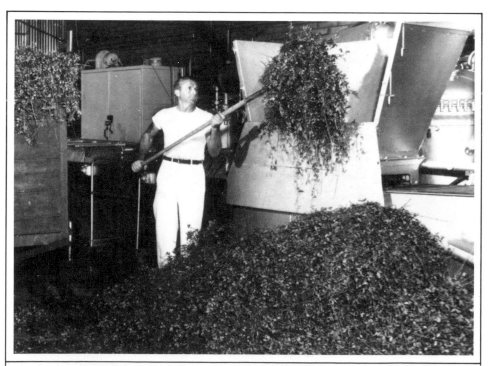

Some nutritional supplements are made from chemical compounds, others from natural ingredients. Here, a worker forks fresh alfalfa into a hopper, where it will be washed, dehydrated and pressed into tablets.

Vitamins and Cancer

Vitamins A, C and E are often mentioned in connection with cancer. The association of cancer with low levels of vitamin A have been reported in an appreciable number of studies. One study showed that for at least twelve months prior to the diagnosis of cancer, vitamin A levels were significantly reduced. Remarkable findings such as these recently prompted the American Cancer Society to publish dietary guidelines that recommended consumption of foods high in vitamin A and related carotenoids (chemicals similar to vitamin A in structure and effect). These are highly concentrated in carrots, tomatoes, broccoli and other yellow and dark-green vegetables.

In animal studies, vitamin A has been shown to provide some degree of protection against the effects of carcinogens, and to postpone or even prevent the development of carci-

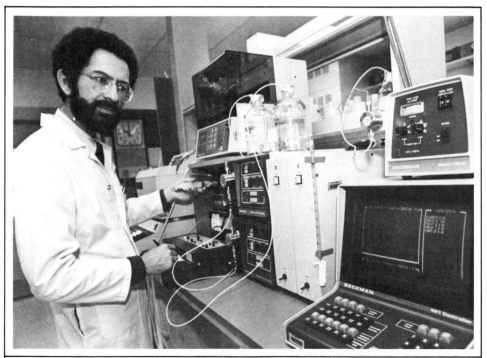

A medical researcher demonstrates the operation of a high-performance liquid chromatograph, a device capable of analyzing the way different vitamins affect the body at different ages.

nomas. Unfortunately, the amounts of vitamin A required to be effective (100,000 IU–150,000 IU daily) are also toxic. Other studies have shown no differences in vitamin A and the carotenoid levels between groups of subjects who developed cancer and those who did not.

Vitamins C and E have also been advocated as prophylactics against cancer, based on the finding that both can prevent or at least delay the formation of carcinomas. They inhibit oxidation, and are therefore specifically suited to prevent the development of cancer-causing nitrosamines in the gut. The incidence of gastrointestinal cancer is highly correlated with the formation of nitrosamines; consequently both vitamins have the potential to help reduce its occurrence.

Spurred by such reports, certain proponents of megavitamin therapy have been encouraging the use of very

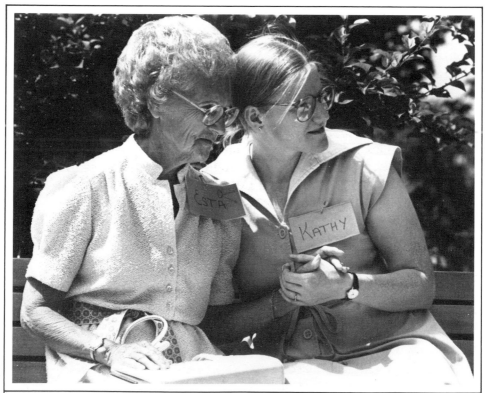

A social worker assists an Alzheimer's disease patient at a community outing. Initial findings show that lecithin and choline alleviate some of the symptoms associated with this disease, though no cure exists.

large amounts of these vitamins, such as daily doses of 10 gm—30 gm of vitamin C for prevention. All in all, more evidence is still required before a final, conclusive statement can be made regarding mega-vitamin treatment as an effective prophylactic against cancer.

Lecithin and Choline

Much is being made of the initial favourable reports of the effects of lecithin and choline on Alzheimer's disease (AD) patients. Present in Alzheimer's disease is a dysfunction (specifically a decreased function) of the cholinergic system (i.e., the neurons and nerves that utilize the neurotransmitter acetylcholine [ACh]). When choline is given to these patients, the body converts it to ACh, and some of the symptoms associated with this disease are alleviated to a certain extent.

Lecithin is simply a large organic molecule known as a *phospholipid* that contains the choline molecule. So the ingestion of either choline or lecithin produces the same effects in the brain and body. Both substances produce some modest, but short-lived improvement in the behaviour of AD patients.

These encouraging findings have been used by certain companies to popularize lecithin and choline as "wonder drugs" capable of producing significant improvements in a healthy person's memory. Furthermore they are lauded as being effective protectors against other types of degenerative dementias. Again, more evidence is needed to substantiate these claims.

Monosodium Glutamate and the Chinese Restaurant Syndrome

In 1968 a Chinese physician named Robert Ho Man Kwok arrived in the United States. He had been told that there were many Chinese restaurants in America, and was very pleased when he discovered that there were even more than he had suspected. His initial enthusiasm was soon dampened—whenever he ate in one he became ill. He usually experienced burning, tightness and numbness in his upper arms, chest, neck and face. This would start soon after he began eating, and sometimes these symptoms would persist for up to four hours.

Dr. Kwok was not the only one who suffered from the Chinese Restaurant Syndrome (CRS). Apparently, anything from two to twenty-five per cent of the population (depending on the study from which the figures are taken) is prone to this phenomenon. In some people, eating in a Chinese restaurant has also been associated with headaches, dizziness, palpitation, general weakness, nausea and vomiting. According to the latest data, headache and nausea seem to be the most common symptoms of CRS, which is primarily caused by the ingestion of monosodium glutamate, or MSG (the salt form of the amino acid glutamic acid).

Cooks in the Far East have used the seaweed *Laminaria japonica* as a flavour enhancer for many years. In 1908 it was discovered that MSG was the substance responsible for the flavour enhancement. With this discovery began the commercial production of MSG throughout the world. In 1984 the worldwide MSG industry produced approximately 300,000 tonnes per year. MSG production and marketing is controlled only by supply and demand. In general MSG must be listed with the ingredients of packaged foods, though for some reason packages of fresh chicken, mayonnaise and salad dressing are not required to list it. MSG is also used extensively as a meat tenderizer.

The initial 1968 report by Dr. Kwok prompted much research into the exact nature and causes of the CRS. Based on the first wave of studies, it was believed that in those people sensitive to MSG, less than 3 gm were needed to produce the characteristic syndrome. It was also shown that even nonsusceptible individuals would manifest the characteristic symptoms if given sufficiently high levels of MSG.

Certain methodological hurdles have, however, been encountered with even the most rigorously controlled double-blind studies. The main problem is that people who are prone to the more uncomfortable effects of MSG are also able to detect its taste, no matter how well concealed it seems to be. Even people who are not prone to its negative effects have been known to discern its unique taste no matter in what type of food it is concealed. Thus in this case the double-blind design fails.

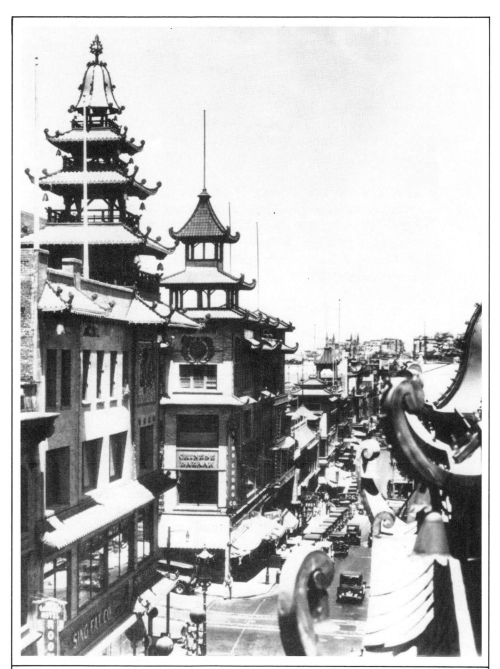

Restaurants in San Francisco's Chinatown (above) and other U.S. cities contribute to the annual national use of about 20,000 tons of monosodium glutamate, or MSG, a flavour enhancer with serious side effects.

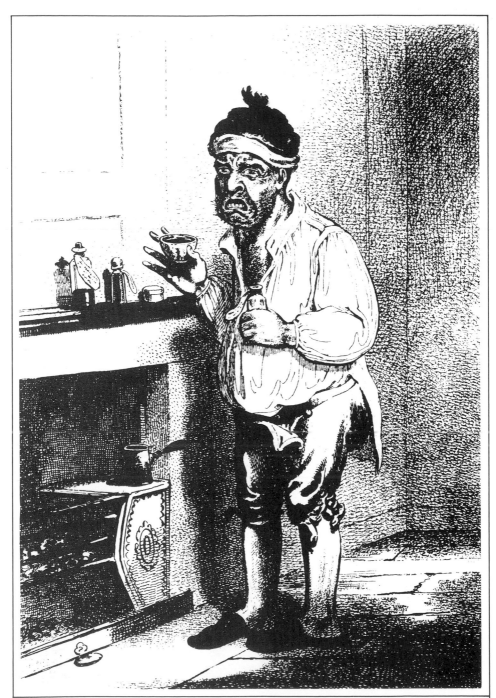

An unhappy headache-sufferer ingests a bitter-tasting "physic" in a cartoon published in 1800. People have used medicine to purge themselves of their aches and pains since before recorded history.

CHAPTER 8

"DO I REALLY NEED THIS?"

At some time in the near future you will go to the medicine cabinet in search of an OTC product for one ailment or another. And the chances are very good that this drug will provide some relief. Yet, many of these OTC products are not considered safe and effective for the disorders for which they are usually intended. What if you used a product not considered effective, but insisted that it gave relief? Aside from the placebo effect, whereby one obtains relief only because the desire and belief that the drug will provide it is strong, there are two other reasons why people often get better when taking OTC drugs.

> *First, most of the diseases for which self-medication is appropriate are so-called self-limiting diseases, like the cold, which get better no matter what you do. Second, many of the products with ingredients lacking evidence of effectiveness do have at least one effective ingredient. So if your symptoms respond quickly, even sooner than if the problem ran its natural course, it is probably due to that ingredient, such as aspirin or paracetamol in a multiple ingredient pain-relief product. The other, ineffective ingredients are not only costing you additional money but are also exposing you to unneeded risks.*
>
> from *Over the Counter Pills that Don't Work*

It is this "additional money" for the pharmaceutical industry which helps keep the products that contain unproven ingredients on the OTC market. Without these ingredients on the market there would be fewer OTC products, and profits would be diminished for the drug industry. If people shop wisely, money can be saved and potential health risks can be decreased. When looking for an OTC product, decide on the most effective ingredient and purchase the product in generic form.

Before you reach for an OTC drug, however, ask yourself this question first: "Do I really need this?" Many symptoms, such as coughs or runny noses, are important in the body's defence against diseases such as the common cold or flu. If the discomfort is not unbearable, it is possible the problem will go away more quickly without the drug. Learn how the body works and how you can help your body heal itself without drugs. Should you decide to take an OTC product, remember that even though it is available without a prescription or the advice of a doctor, it can be dangerous. Whether you purchased it from a pharmacy or not, it should be used only when needed and with caution.

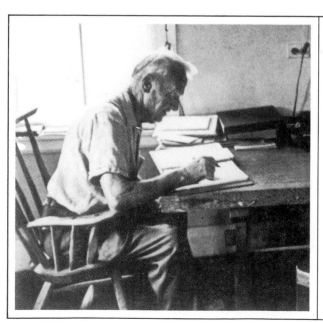

Scott Nearing, American author of Living the Good Life, *lived with his wife in rural Maine, where they grew all their food and bartered for those commodities they were unable to produce. Eating organically-grown foods and getting regular physical exercise, he avoided all medicines and doctors and remained healthy until he died in 1984, two weeks before his 100th birthday.*

Some Useful Addresses

In the United Kingdom:

Advisory Council on the Misuse of Drugs
c/o Home Office, Queen Anne's Gate, London SW1H 9AT.

British Association for Counselling
87a Sheep Street, Rugby, Warwicks CV21 3BX.

Department of Education and Science
Elizabeth House, York Road, London SE1 7PH.

Health Education Council
78 New Oxford Street, London WC1A 1AH.

Home Office Drugs Branch
Queen Anne's Gate, London SW1H 9AT.

Institute for the Study of Drug Dependence
1–4 Hatton Place, Hatton Garden, London EC1N 8ND.

Medical Research Council
20 Park Crescent, London W1N 4AL.

Narcotics Anonymous
PO Box 246, c/o 47 Milman Street, London SW10.

National Association of Young People's Counselling
and Advisory Services
17–23 Albion Street, Leicester LE1 6GD.

Northern Ireland Department of Health and Social Services
Upper Newtownwards Road, Belfast BT4 3SF.

Release
1 Elgin Avenue, London W9.

Scottish Health Education Unit
21 Lansdowne Crescent, Edinburgh EH12 5EH.

Scottish Home and Health Department
St. Andrews House, Edinburgh EH1 3DE.

Some Useful Addresses

Standing Conference on Drug Abuse
1–4 Hatton Place, Hatton Garden, London EC1N 8ND.

Teachers Advisory Council on Alcohol and Drug Education
2 Mount Street, Manchester M2 5NG.

In Australia:

Department of Health
PO Box 100, Wooden ACT, Australia 2606.

In New Zealand:

Drug Advisory Committee
Department of Health, PO Box 5013, Wellington.

Drug Dependence
11–23 Sturdee Street, Wellington.

Drug Dependency Clinic
393 Great North Road, Grey Lynn, Auckland.

Medical Services and Drug Control
Department of Health, PO Box 5013, Wellington.

National Drug Intelligence Bureau
Police Department, Private Bag, Wellington.

In South Africa:

South African National Council on Alcoholism
and Drug Dependence (SANCA) National Office
PO Box 10134, Johannesburg 2000.

A number of organizations in South Africa provide information and services in the field of drug dependence. SANCA will supply information on these, as will the government's Department of Health and Welfare.

Further Reading

Alhadeff, L., Gualtieri, T., and Lipton, M. "Toxic effects of water-soluble vitamins". *Nutrition Reviews* vol. 42 (1984): pp. 33–40.

Allen, D.M., Greenblatt, D.J., and Noel, B.J. "Self-poisoning with over-the-counter hypnotics". *Clinical Toxicology* vol. 15 (1979): pp. 151–158.

Beaver, W.T. "Caffeine revisited". *Journal of the American Medical Association* vol. 251 (1984): pp.1732–1733.

Benowicz, Robert J. *Non-Prescription Drugs & Their Side Effects*. New York: Putnam Publishing Group, 1983.

Blum, A. "Phenylpropanolamine: An over-the-counter amphetamine?" *Journal of the American Medical Association* vol. 245 (1981): pp. 1346–1347.

Cawood, F.W. and Smith, D.C. *Vitamin Side Effects Revealed*. Peachtree City, Georgia: F.C. and A. Publishing, 1984.

Esmay, J.B. and Wertheimer, A.I. "A review of over-the-counter drug therapy". *Journal of Community Health* vol. 5 (1979): pp. 54–66.

Griffith, H. Winter. *Complete Guide to Prescription & Non-Prescription Drugs*. Tucson: HPBooks, 1985.

Kaufman, J., Rabinowitz-Dagi, L., Levin, J., McCarthy, P., Wolfe, S., Bargmann, E., and The Public Citizen Health Research Group. *Over-the-Counter Pills that Don't Work*. New York: Pantheon, 1983.

Ritter, R.M. "PPA: diet drug under fire". *Psychology Today* vol. 18 (1984): pp. 8–12.

Vener, A.M., Krupka, L.R., and Climo, J.J. "Drugs (prescription, over-the-counter, social) and the young adult: use and attitudes". *The International Journal of Addiction* vol. 17 (1982): pp. 399–415.

Wooliscroft, J.O. "Megavitamins: fact and fancy". *Disease-A-Month* vol. 29 (1983): pp. 1–56.

Glossary

acetylsalicylic acid   aspirin; an analgesic and antipyretic

addiction   a condition caused by repeated drug use, including a compulsive urge to continue using the drug, a tendency to increase the dosage, and physiological and/or psychological dependence

adenosine   a neurotransmitter affected by caffeine

adjuvant   a drug used to enhance the effects of another drug

adrenal gland   a gland located near the kidney that produces the hormone adrenaline (also known as epinephrine) used in the treatment of asthma

adulterate   to dilute a drug either with an inert material to add bulk or another drug to alter the effects of the original drug

alkaloid   any chemical containing nitrogen, carbon, hydrogen and oxygen, usually occurring in plants

allergic response   the body's reaction to infected, damaged or disturbed tissue, characterized by inflammation, sneezing, congestion, runny nose and/or watery, itchy, red eyes

Alzheimer's disease   a dysfunction (specifically a decreased function) of the cholinergic system, characterized by a loss of memory and/or judgment and often accompanied by confusion

analgesic   a drug that produces an insensitivity to pain without loss of consciousness

anorectic   an appetite suppressant

anticholinergic   a drug that alters the normal communication between neurons by binding to the receptor sites normally used by the neurotransmitter acetylcholine (ACh)

antihistamine   a drug that inhibits the action of histamine and thus reduces the allergic response

anti-inflammatory   a drug that reduces inflammation

antipyretic   a drug that reduces fever

antitussive   substances that act to inhibit an uncontrollable, dry or unproductive cough

aspirin   acetylsalicylic acid; an analgesic, antipyretic

and anti-inflammatory agent originally derived from plants

asthma   a condition characterized by a difficulty in breathing, often caused by constriction of the bronchi of the lungs and treated with epinephrine-related drugs

atherosclerosis   a degenerative disease of the arteries

atropine   an anticholinergic drug extracted from the belladonna plant and used to relieve spasms, to diminish secretions, to relieve pain, and to dilate the pupil

autism   a psychological condition characterized by mental activity which is controlled by the wishes of the individuals as opposed to mental activity controlled by the conditions imposed by the nature of objects and events

axon   the part of a neuron along which the nerve impulse travels away from the cell body

barbiturate   a drug that causes depression of the central nervous system, generally used to reduce anxiety or to induce euphoria

belladonna   the deadly nightshade; a plant from which many anticholinergics are derived

benzodiazepine   a potent reliever of anxiety and insomnia; includes Valium and Librium

"black beauties"   black-market amphetamines

bronchodilator   a substance that, by dilating the bronchi of the lungs, clears the air passages and aids breathing

buffer   a substance that lowers acidity; sometimes added to aspirin to decrease this drug's irritation to the stomach

caffeine   trimethylxanthine; a central nervous system stimulator found in coffee, tea, cocoa, various soft drinks, and often in combination with other drugs to enhance their effects

carcinogen   a substance that causes the formation of carcinomas which lead to cancer

cardiac arrhythmias   irregular beating of the heart

cataract   a clouding of the lens of the eye

catecholamines   neurotransmitters such as epinephrine and dopamine

CAT scan   an x-ray technique that produces x-ray

photographs of a part of the body from any cross-section or angle

cholinergic system   the neurons and nerves that utilize the neurotransmitter acetylcholine (ACh)

codeine   a sedative and pain-relieving agent found in opium and related to morphine but less potent

coenzyme   a nonprotein compound that forms the active portion of an enzyme system

collagen   a protein found in bone, cartilage and connective tissue and involved in the process of healing

dendrites   hair-like structures protruding from the neural cell body on which receptor sites are located

dextromethorphan   an antitussive

diabetes mellitus   a disorder caused by an inadequate secretion or utilization of insulin and characterized by thirst, hunger, itching, weakness, loss of weight and, when severe, coma

dilation   the action of stretching or expanding an organ or part of the body

DNA   deoxyribonucleic acid; the substance found in the cell nucleus and associated with the transmission of genetic information

dopamine   a form of dopa, an amino acid used in the treatment of Parkinson's disease, and found in the adrenal gland

double-blind study   an experimental design used in testing the effectiveness of drugs which compares the drug in question with a placebo and, to obtain objective results, maintains both the subject's and the drug administrator's ignorance of the actual content of the substance ingested by the subject

endorphins   chemicals found in the brain and recognized as the body's own painkillers, acting in a manner similar to morphine and codeine

ephedrine   a bronchodilator whose actions relax smooth muscles, stimulate the heart and the central nervous system, and constrict the blood vessels

epinephrine   a sympathomimetic drug used in the emergency treatment of severe allergic reactions, especially to insect stings

euphoria   a mental high characterized by a sense of well-being *expectorant* a substance that facilitates or promotes the discharge of mucus from the respiratory tract accumulated during the common cold or flu

fibrocystic breast disease an abnormal increase of fibrous connective tissue in the breast

glaucoma an eye disease characterized by increased pressure within the eye which ultimately leads to blindness

haemorrhage to bleed

hepatitis inflammation of the liver, often associated with the use of contaminated hypodermic needles

hepatotoxic causing damage to the liver

histamine a chemical found in all body tissues that serves both as a neurotransmitter in the brain and as an important agent in inflammation and allergic reactions

hyperlipemia an excess of fat or lipids in the blood

hypertension high blood pressure

ibuprofen an analgesic, anti-inflammatory and anti-pyretic drug

International Unit a quantity of a biological substance, such as a vitamin, that produces a particular biological effect agreed upon internationally

ischaemic attacks localized tissue anaemia due to decreased blood supply

macrophage specialized cells, present at the site of inflammation, which get rid of unwanted foreign substances and dead tissue

methapyrilene an antihistamine previously combined with scopolamine and used as a sleep aid

myocardial infarction heart muscle degeneration due to inadequate blood flow

narcotic originally, a group of drugs producing effects similar to morphine; often used to refer to any substance that sedates, has a depressive effect and/or causes dependence

nephrolithiasis a condition characterized by having gall stones

neuron a specialized cell, composed of a cell body, axons and dendrites, which carries electrical messages and is the structural unit of the nervous system

neurosis a psychological disorder which originates as a

mental condition, though it may come to include physiological symptoms

neurotransmitter a chemical, such as ACh, that travels from the axon of one neuron, across the synaptic gap, and to the receptor site on the dendrite of an adjacent neuron, thus allowing communication between neural cells

nitrosamines compounds that can produce cancer in the stomach

nucleotides substances important in the formation of DNA and RNA

orthomolecular psychiatry a type of therapy for mental illness that includes diets centred around mega-doses of multiple vitamins and minerals

paracetamol N-acetylpara-amino-phenol, or APAP; a potent analgesic and antipyretic chemically similar to aspirin yet without anti-inflammatory action

paranoid schizophrenia a mental disorder characterized by persistent delusions, often with hallucinations

peripheral vascular occlusion the closing of superficial blood vessels, usually those supplying the legs

pernicious anaemia a disorder that prevents the absorption of vitamin B_{12} into the blood stream

phenacetin an analgesic related to paracetamol

phenylisopropylamine a class of drugs which contains amphetamine, ephedrine, and PPA

phenylpropanolamine (PPA) a sympathomimetic drug with anorectic action

phospholipid a class of large organic molecules found in all living cells in association with fats; includes lecithin

physical dependence an adaptation of the body to the presence of a drug, such that its absence produces withdrawal symptoms

placebo effect a pharmacologic effect on a symptom produced by a substance either pharmacologically inert or active only in the treatment of unrelated symptoms

premenstrual syndrome a syndrome which occurs prior to a woman's menstrual period and is characterized by fluid retention, sensitive or painful breasts, and irritability

prophylactic something that helps to prevent disease

prostaglandins chemicals released within the body during inflammation

prostate gland a gland that surrounds the male uretha into which it secretes a lubricating fluid

psychological dependence a condition in which the drug user craves a drug to maintain a sense of well-being and feels discomfort when deprived of it

psychotic behaviour abnormal or pathological behaviour which includes the loss of contact with reality and occasionally hallucinations and delusions

rebound congestion a condition that occurs when, after discontinuing use of a decongestant, the congestion becomes worse than it was initially

receptor sites specialized areas located on dendrites which, when bound by a sufficient number of neurotransmitter molecules, produce an electrical charge

rheumatoid arthritis a disease characterized by inflammation and swelling of the joints and often leading to stiffening and permanent disability

RNA a substance found in the cell and associated with the control of cellular chemical activities

salicylates a family of pain relievers containing salicylic acid derived from plants

scopolamine an anticholinergic with sedative, analgesic qualities, previously included in antihistamines

scurvy a disease caused by a lack of vitamin C and characterized by weakness, spongy gums, anaemia, and bleeding gums and other mucous membranes

speed amphetamine

stroke a condition caused by the bursting of a blood vessel in the brain and the resultant death of that part of the brain deprived of its blood supply

sympathetic nervous system a system of nerves which, during an emergency, elicits responses of alertness, excitement and alarm, and controls the expenditure of necessary energy

sympathomimetic drug a drug that produces effects which mimic those produced by the sympathetic nervous system

synaptic gap the space between the axon and dendrite of two neurons in which neurotransmitters travel *synergism*　when two drugs together produce effects greater than either one alone

thrombophlebitis:　inflammation of a vein associated with, or due to, a thrombus, or blood clot

tolerance　a decrease of susceptibility to the effects of a drug due to its continued administration, resulting in the user's need to increase the drug dosage in order to achieve the effects experienced previously

topical drug　a drug designed for local application, such as in the form of inhalants, sprays or drops

uppers　amphetamines

vasodilation　dilation of a blood vessel

venous thrombosis:　clotting of the blood in a vein

withdrawal　the physiological and psychological effects of discontinued usage of a drug

xanthines　a class of drugs derived from the compound xanthine which naturally occurs in plants and is a central nervous system stimulant

Index

Index

Index

Paul Sanberg, Ph. D., an assistant professor of psychology and bio-medical sciences at Ohio University, received his degree from the Australian National University in Canberra. He was a visiting scholar in the neuroscience department at the University of California and a post-doctorial fellow in the departments of Neuroscience and psychiatry at The Johns Hopkins Medical School.

Richard M. T. Krema received his B.A. in psychology from Laurentian University, Ontario, and is currently a graduate student in behavioural neuroscience at Ohio University.

Solomon H. Snyder, M.D., is Distinguished Service Professor of Neuroscience, Pharmacology and Psychiatry at The Johns Hopkins University School of Medicine. He has served as president of the Society for Neuroscience and in 1978 received the Albert Laster Award in Medical Research. He is the author of *Uses of Marijuana, Madness and the Brain, The Troubled Mind, Biological Aspects of Mental Disorder,* and edited *Perspective in Neuropharmacology: A Tribute to Julius Axelrod.* Professor Snyder was a research associate with Dr. Axelrod at the National Institute of Health.

Malcolm Lader, D.Sc., Ph.D., M.D., F.R.C. Psych. is Professor of Clinical Psychopharmacology at the Institute of Psychiatry, University of London, and Honorary Consultant to the Bethlem Royal and Maudsley Hospitals. He is a member of the External Scientific Staff of the Medical Research Council. He has researched extensively into the actions of drugs used to treat psychiatric illnesses and symptoms, in particular the tranquillizers. He has written several books and over 300 scientific articles. Professor Lader is a member of several governmental advisory committees concerned with drugs.

Paul Williams, M.B., M.R.C., Psych., D.P.M., is Senior Lecturer at the Institute of Psychiatry, University of London, Deputy Director of the General Practice research Unit and Honorary Consultant Psychiatrist at the Bethlem Royal and Maudsley Hospitals. His research has been largely concerned with the extent of psychiatric disorder in the community, and its management in general practice. Within this field, his particular interest has been in investigating the extent and patterns of use of psychotropic drugs.